Praise for BurnoutRx® for

Healthcare Professionals

Dr. Strich has written a clear, concise and practical guide to assessing, preventing and recovering from burnout for healthcare professionals. Based on his personal experience and the growing research literature, Dr. Strich offers a roadmap for the healthcare team to follow to address the costly (economic and psychological) problem of burnout among all members of the healthcare team. Written from the perspective of a professional coach to individuals, groups and healthcare systems this is a book that should be read and re-read by all members of the healthcare community

Dennis Greenberger, Ph.D.

Mind Over Mood, Co-author

Director, Anxiety and Depression Center

Newport Beach, California

Dr Gideon Strich is a critical thinker with a heart and soul. He shares important ideas on how to manage burnout based onresearch and "me-search." He experienced serious burnout and recovered. His journey is inspiring. His research and tips are important and very helpful. If you have ever worried about how well your work is a good fit for your values and beliefs and life satisfaction, you will be well served with Dr Strich's suggestions for self-exploration.

Sharon Livingston, Ph.D.

Director, The Livingston Center for Professional Coaching

New York, N.Y.

BurnoutRx®

For Healthcare Professionals

Gideon Strich, M.D.

The information in this volume is not intended as a substitute for consultation with healthcare professionals. Each individual's health concerns should be evaluated by a qualified professional.

Purchasers of this book have permission to copy worksheets and boxes for personal use only. No other part of this book may be reproduced, translated, stored in a retrieval system, or transmitted, in any form or by any means, electronic, mechanical, photocopying, microfilming, recording, or otherwise, without written permission from the publisher.

Printed in the United States of America

ISBN: 9781671989863

DEDICATION

This book is dedicated to the men and women on the front lines of healthcare delivery, trying to mend broken people while working in a broken healthcare system.

CONTENTS

ACKNOWLEDGMENTS

I would like to acknowledge the excellent training I received in coaching and NLP from Dr. Sharon Livingston, Dr. Jeffrey Auerbach and Dr. Matt James without whom I would not be enjoying my new career as a coach.

INTRODUCTION

This book grew out of my own experience with physician burnout, my years of working on a hospital physician well-being committee and my experience coaching physicians and other healthcare professionals. This year I started coaching medical students. Working with the medical students was eye-opening because they and the current crop of residents are in the first group of Millenials to enter mainstream medicine. Unlike their Boomer and Gen-x predecessors they dislike being lectured to and prefer to get their learning in an interactive online format. They also have a different world view and set of expectations, especially regarding work-life balance. While they are just as intelligent, motivated and compassionate as their predecessors, many expect to be employees when they graduate and view medicine as a job rather than an avocation.

My purpose in writing this book was to share some of the knowledge and practices that I used to recover from physician burnout, in the hopes that I could help someone else faced with the same challenge. After I recovered, I did extensive research into the causes and prevention of burnout in health care professions. I realized that I needed to speak to *all* of the healthcare professions that interact in the inpatient and outpatient environments—including physicians, nurses, therapists, social workers and even managers and executives. The reason is because none of us work alone. Healthcare is always delivered in teams, and the team simply does not function well if one or one or more of its members are burned out. So even though the book is written from a physician's perspective, the lessons and exercises apply to all of the health care professionals working as a team in these environments.

Once I had recovered, I looked for a way to remain involved in healthcare so that I could have a positive impact on both providers and patients. That search led me to discover the profession of coaching, and I went on to take two years of coach training. Following my training and certification, I decided to coach specifically in the area of burnout prevention and recovery. In addition to coaching individual healthcare providers, I also aimed to bring coaching to medical students since many of the conditions and mindsets that lead to professional burnout are established during medical school. I view early intervention in the form of medical student coaching as being analogous to vaccination against burnout. It is more beneficial to prevent a condition than to try to treat It after it occurs. For that reason I ran a pilot project for first-year medical students consisting of a series of 12 one-hour online group coaching sessions that contained equal parts of didactic material and experiential exercises. This book's structure and some of the exercises contained herein are distilled from that experience.

The subtitle of the book is *"10 things you can do today to prevent or recover from burnout."* That's because there are 10 chapters corresponding to 10 categories of actions. However, if you read the book in its entirety, you will notice that each chapter contains several specific actions that you can take. So, the subtitle is a little bit misleading in that I don't expect you to complete all of the actions *today*. The important takeaway from this message is that you can **begin** at least one of them – and then build from there.

Chapter 1

WHY YOU HATE YOUR JOB

W e've all heard the phrase before, but the fact that it's become so widely used doesn't make it any less accurate: more and more people are feeling *burned out*. And, it's especially rampant in the healthcare industry. You might be one of these people, but also might be hesitant to use this label for your situation. So how do you truly know if this applies to you? Consider the following three questions; if you can answer yes to any one of the three, you are most likely either burned out or on your way.

1. Do you come home exhausted after work most days and don't feel quite recharged the next day -- even after getting 8 hours of sleep?

2. Do you find yourself making cynical remarks or having negative thoughts about some of your patients or clients?

3. Do you wonder whether what you're doing is actually *helping* anyone, especially yourself?

The truth is if you feel "burned out" on a regular basis, you probably are. Since about 50% of physicians and a similar proportion of hospital nurses are burned out statistically, the assumption that you're in this group is likely to be right. But how can you really know for sure?

There are some commonly used objective measures of burnout. The gold standard is the Maslach Burnout inventory—a 22 question, self-scored survey that divides people into categories of low-level, moderate, and high-level burnout. This was the measure that most burnout research used until about five years ago, when Mayo Clinic developed the Well-being Index. This nine-element survey reports measures of likelihood of burnout, meaning in work, fatigue, work-life integration, risk for medical error, and suicidal ideation. There are now separate indices for nurses and medical students as well.

Try this: Below is an abbreviated form of the Maslach Burnout Inventory.

How to Score: Add up all the numbers corresponding to your circles. While this survey is not as precise as the full Maslach, you can estimate your risk as follows:

<10 low risk for burnout -Even though you aren't burned out now, read through the rest of the book to see how you can prevent burnout in the future.

10-20 moderate risk for burnout- Continue reading and try one or more of the recommended interventions to improve your quality of life

>20 high risk for burnout- Get on it right away. Get a coach (or therapist if you're clinically depressed) and work through the exercises beginning with mindfulness, before you cause yourself (or someone else) further suffering.

You can re-take this survey at any time to see how much progress you're making, or you might try the Well-being Index at:

https://www.mywellbeingindex.org/

Circle each number that applies to you for each question on this worksheet

	Never	A few times a year	Once a month or less	A few times a month	Once a week	A few times a week	Every day
I feel emotionally drained from my work	0	1	2	3	4	5	6
I feel fatigued when I get up in the morning and have to face another day	0	1	2	3	4	5	6
Working with people all day is a strain for me	0	1	2	3	4	5	6
I feel I treat some patients/clients as if they were impersonal objects	0	1	2	3	4	5	6
I've become more callous toward people since I took this job	0	1	2	3	4	5	6
I really don't care what happens to some patients/clients	0	1	2	3	4	5	6
I deal very effectively with the problems of my patients/clients	6	5	4	3	2	1	0
I feel I am positively influencing other people's lives through my work	6	5	4	3	2	1	0
I feel exhilarated after working closely with my patients/clients	6	5	4	3	2	1	0

So now that we know where you are, let's define what burnout really is – so you can start taking steps toward prevention and if needed, recovery.

What *is* burnout?

The concept of occupational related burnout was first described by psychologist Christina Maslach back in 1981. More recently, the World Health Organization added occupational burnout to the ICD-11 (International Classification of Diseases) diagnostic manual. According to the WHO,

---

"Burnout is a syndrome conceptualized as resulting from chronic workplace stress that has not been successfully managed. It is characterized by three dimensions:

1. Feelings of energy depletion or exhaustion;

2. Increased mental distance from one's job, or feelings of negativism or cynicism related to one's job; and

3. Reduced professional efficacy.

Burn-out refers specifically to phenomena in the occupational context and should not be applied to describe experiences in other areas of life."

Burnout among physicians and other healthcare professionals really wasn't recognized until about 10 to 12 years ago when the first studies from Mayo clinic were published. Initial studies of physicians, from about 10 years ago, demonstrated a burnout rate of approximately 45% using the Maslach criteria. That amount is *almost double* that found in other working adults. Those numbers became particularly disturbing when research was done documenting both the personal and professional consequences of burnout among healthcare professionals.

Professionally, burned out physicians make more medical mistakes, have less satisfied and compliant patients, have a higher risk of drug or alcohol abuse, may exhibit disruptive behavior in the workplace, and are more likely to leave medical practice. On a personal level, it was found that burnout correlated with increased depression, anxiety, relationship problems, and most importantly, a higher risk of completed suicide.

It is important to recognize that women may experience and express burnout differently than men. A 2018 Medscape survey of more than 15,000 physicians showed that female physicians reported burnout more often than male physicians (48% vs. 38%.) Additionally, more than half of women discussed it with family and friends vs. 39% for men. Women tend to report physical and emotional exhaustion first, followed by depersonalization and cynicism, and a feeling of loss of efficacy and increased self-doubt. Men tend to express cynicism and anger first, followed by emotional exhaustion. They are often in denial about loss of efficacy, although their co-workers and patients may report this.

Men and women also cope with burnout differently. Women were more likely to sleep more, eat junk food and binge eat, whereas men were more likely to use exercise to cope. Most importantly, women were more likely to seek professional help than men (31% vs. 24%.) My hope—and in fact, one of the reasons I wrote this book—is that as burnout and its causes become better understood and de-stigmatized, more physicians will seek the help they need either through counseling or coaching.

The economic consequences of burnout have also recently been quantified. The estimated cost of replacing a primary care physician in the United States is approximately $900,000. This includes the cost of recruitment, training, and lost productivity associated with the turnover. That cost for nurses is approximately $150,000 to $200,000. A 2019 article in the Annals of Internal Medicine put the cost of physician burnout to the economy at *4.2 billion dollars per year* in terms of lost productivity. That does not include the costs of decreased patient outcomes and increased malpractice costs associated with burnout.

My Burnout Story

Before we delve into the causes of burnout, I'd like to share my own burnout story here. Even now, five years after retiring from active clinical practice, I find it incredibly difficult to tell this story. Not only does it require me to recount a very sad and difficult chapter of my life; but despite everything I'm going to tell you in the following pages, there's still a lingering feeling in the back of my mind (that I know is not true) that this was somehow a personal failure. However, I know that it wasn't a failure, of any sort; in getting through it and sharing my story to help others, I'm hoping to change that feeling to one of accomplishment. I will also share with you the positive aspects of burnout (yes – there are some!), and the importance of bringing it out in the open and sharing it with your peers.

For 30 years, I was a practicing diagnostic and interventional radiologist and worked both in an outpatient office and an inpatient setting in a very busy metropolitan trauma center. As you can imagine, there was a lot of time and performance stress associated with this job, since many of our patients came in through the emergency room or following significant trauma and required an immediate response from the radiology department.

Over time, my medical group evolved from a group with whom I had shared values to a younger group with whom I did not share the same hierarchy of values. Over that period of 25 years, I had four or five episodes of burnout, which is (sadly) fairly typical for a busy physician. I felt exhausted, unmotivated, and almost crushed by the responsibility of the job and of providing for a family. Somehow, like all physicians, I soldiered on; and after a period of months, became fully functional again.

The final episode of burnout—the one that ended my career—occurred when I was 59. It resulted from a confluence of events, a "perfect storm" of stressors. Our medical group had gone through some difficult financial times. Consequently, we decided to sell the practice to a national corporation. This resulted in a change of leadership—one that, in my opinion, was not a change for the better. There was a sense among the physicians, as well as the staff, of loss of control. There was a gradual erosion in the rapport and the quality of interaction between the physicians and staff, which led to a more hostile working environment for everyone.

At the same time, my marriage of 30 years had failed. I was separated and going through a very contentious divorce. I recognized that I was very depressed and sought out professional help; but even that couldn't prevent my slide down the slippery slope of burnout. I was having a harder and harder time maintaining my focus and doing the challenging cognitive work my profession required.

The final straw came on a week when one of my partners went on vacation and I was asked to cover his work as well as my own. On the second day of that week, I found myself sitting in front of four computer monitors with thousands of images on them, struggling to make any kind of sense of what I was doing or seeing. The kind of interpretation which had previously seemed challenging but doable now seemed beyond comprehension. At that moment, my whole world just seemed to *stop*. I put down my Dictaphone, walked out of my office, closed the door, and went home. At that moment, all I really wanted was to get away from the stress and the pain. I fully intended to take a large dose of benzodiazepines and drink myself into oblivion.

However, I decided to call my girlfriend when I got home and tell her of my plans, mostly because I had a tremendous amount of guilt about the effect it would have on her. Quite wisely, she left work and came over to my house and convinced me to let her take me to a hospital that had a specialized inpatient unit. I was admitted for a couple of days and then released into a partial outpatient program for the next five months until I was no longer suicidal.

I then took another six months off while I was recovering. Following that, I considered going back to work. But when I approached my group, they had decided that my depression was a medicolegal

7

liability for the group, and therefore terminated my employment. Of course, I was initially devastated. Not only did my livelihood depend on my ability to practice medicine; my identity for the last 30 years had been closely tied to my practice and my professional accomplishments.

The story *does* have a happy ending, though. After a year of trying to find myself and my place in the world, I discovered the profession of coaching. I spent about two years taking classes in professional and executive coaching before deciding to dedicate myself to coaching healthcare professionals going through or at risk for burnout.

In the following chapters, I will share with you not only the best practices of coaching that I learned through my training and mentorship, but also the lessons that I've learned in my experience coaching healthcare professionals, and more recently, medical students. I will briefly touch on the causes of burnout in healthcare and provide you with a framework and a clear path to recover from or prevent professional burnout and to live a fulfilling life of purpose and meaning.

What causes burnout?

Author and physician coach Dr. Dike Drummond wrote an excellent article in the September 2015 issue of *Family Practice Management* in which he describes five main causes of burnout.

First is the **nature of the job itself**. Whether you are a physician, or a nurse, or an allied health care practitioner, caring for sick people and their families takes a lot of energy, even when you're doing well. Patients and their families may be upset, demanding, or even abusive; yet it's your job to take care of all patients with an equal amount of energy, skill, and compassion. Although you train for this in medical or nursing school, it's another thing to actually deal with life-and-death situations or bad clinical outcomes. It can be extremely stressful.

Second, there are stressors associated with **your specific job conditions**, including your work hours, your call rotation, the number of patients you're expected to take care of, and the other people in your clinic, practice or hospital unit. Studies have shown that interpersonal conflict is one of the major causes of nurse burnout. Of course, nobody practices alone, and there are many factors associated with your clinic, network, and hospital, including hospital administration. Research speaks to the fact that the rate of burnout in units or organizations with poor leadership is higher than those where leadership is responsive to front-line staff feedback or needs.

Thirdly, there's the element of trying to achieve **work-life balance**. Ideally, a perfectly balanced life would include eight hours at work, eight hours with your family and friends, and eight hours sleeping every day. Can you think of the last time you had a day like this? We know that this rarely happens. Sometimes situations at work require longer hours, and we are conditioned not to say no when our peers request our help—even if we already feel physically and mentally exhausted. This is partially due to the type of personality that people who go into healthcare inherently *have*; another part is due to our training in school or in residency. Alternatively, situations can arise at home that demand more of your time and energy. These demands may come from a spouse, child, parents, or friends. Choosing between spending more time and energy at home or at work causes an internal conflict that contributes to the stress of medical practice. So rather than **work-life balance**, we should aim for **work-life harmony**. Chapter 10 covers this notion and offers tips and exercises for achieving it.

The fourth factor is **our own individual conditioning**. Some of this has to do with the way we were brought up and our family's values. Let's face it: you have to be a hard worker, extremely motivated, and competitive in order to get into medical school. These tendencies toward being a workaholic and perfectionist are only cultivated more during medical education and training.

During my medical training, it was not uncommon for me and my fellow students to work 100 hours a week or more. In fact, we used to say, "the only problem with being on call every other night is that you miss half the good cases!" Fortunately, there are now legal parameters regarding how long a medical student or resident can work—usually 80 hours a week. That's still quite a lot, and some training programs find ways to circumvent that rule. Medical professionals' competitive nature means that we never say no when we're asked to do additional work. We don't want others to see us as "weak"—which also leads to the belief that we should never ask for help. This perfectionism often means that we hold ourselves and everyone around us to an impossible standard, since perfection is impossible to attain. We should strive for *excellence* instead of perfection.

During our medical training, we learn **two habitual thought patterns** that we're often not aware of. One is "the patient always comes first"—which is of course necessary when we're at work. But when we're not at work, we need to learn self-care, a skill that is normally *not* taught in medical school. The other unconscious lesson is "never show weakness." We believe that we have to do everything ourselves and not ask for help, in case we are perceived as weak or less capable. We are like the Lone Ranger, but without Tonto to help us. Because we're not willing to ask for help, it's tempting to keep going even when we're mentally and physically exhausted. This is how we enter the downward spiral of burnout.

The fifth major factor that's relevant to burnout in physicians and nurses is the **quality of leadership**—not only within the work unit, but throughout the institution. If organizational leadership is fully focused on finances and business metrics, it becomes too easy for them to see doctors and nurses as cost centers instead of valuable assets. This often leads to a toxic environment where both doctors and nurses feel that they can't get support from their organizations and don't feel valued. But there are medical organizations that recognize the value of their human assets. Some of them utilize Lean-Sigma management, a management model developed by Toyota Motor Corporation in the 1980's. In this model, the front-line providers lead the way in practice development and the job of the C-suite is to provide the support to make them successful. Having been a patient in such a facility I can tell you it is a very different experience. The staff are cooperative and friendly and as a patient you feel valued and cared for. Interestingly, many of these organizations are more successful financially than those run in a traditional top-down approach, probably due to increased employee engagement.

Dr. Drummond doesn't include in his list of elements the national, state, and business environments in which healthcare workers operate. According to the AMA, these factors account for 75% of burnout drivers. The five factors listed above are 25% of the causes; but this 25% is at least *somewhat* within the individual's control, and therefore what I focus on in this book.

The best and highest use of burnout

You may not believe it but burnout can have positive outcomes. Among other things, the burnout epidemic is bringing needed public awareness to this problem. What is really needed is for healthcare organizations, insurance organizations and political leaders to take concrete action to make the healthcare environment more user friendly for the providers

Going through burnout can also be an opportunity for you to do some serious self-reflection and make needed changes in your life. In the remainder of the book I will introduce you to new information and step-by-step exercises to help you re-evaluate where you are, what you want, and how to get it.

Since you now know where you fall on the burnout spectrum, consider the questions in the following exercise. If you haven't experience burnout as we've defined it, think back to a particularly difficult time or challenge you faced professionally.

In the below exercise, try re-framing your experience and imagining a beneficial outcome for yourself.

Try this:

1. What is your burnout story? Reflect on a time in your career when you have felt burned out, physically and emotionally exhausted by your work.

2. Write down all the details. How did you get to that point? What were the internal and external factors that contributed?

3. If you recovered, what happened to change things? Was it something you or someone else did, or a change in circumstances?

4. Try re-framing the story in a positive way. What did you learn that helps you now or could help you in the future. What positive thing came out of your experience that would not have happened if you didn't go through that experience.

5. Write a new chapter. Imagine that you woke up one morning and a miracle had happened and you were living your ideal life. What would your work situation be like? How about your home or social life? Where would you be? Who would you be with? Fill in all the details and make that vision as real and compelling as you can.

6. With that vision in mind, what is the first thing that has to happen to make that ideal life a reality.

7. Try sharing your story with a friend, or your spouse or a trusted colleague. If you're brave share it anonymously on my website at https://www.gideonstrichmd.com/my-burnout-story/

Burnout is an energy problem.

Like Dr. Drummond, I see burnout as primarily an energy problem. In my conception, we have four different types of energy that we use every day: physical energy, emotional energy, mental energy, and spiritual energy. There's a constant flow of energy between these areas, so that each can support or drain the others. Dr. Drummond likens this to an "energy bank account", where every use of energy at work is like a withdrawal. We can also make deposits into this account. We recharge our energy in various ways, including rest, time off, or positive interactions with co-workers, families and friends. Each time we recharge, we make a deposit into our energy bank account. And just like a bank account, if we continue to withdraw more energy than we deposit, we eventually run into a deficit where our energy account is overdrawn. Like a bank account or credit card, we start accumulating accrued interest, which puts us further into deficit, and eventually leads to the downward spiral of burnout.

Burnout is your mind-body's way of declaring bankruptcy. Fortunately, most people recover from burnout (and bankruptcy) to get a new start, hopefully with some hard-earned lessons. Unfortunately, some don't. Physicians die by suicide at *almost double* the rate of other professionals and the statistics are even worse for women than for men. I will talk more about energy and time management in later chapters; but for now, let's focus on an important aspect of experiencing burnout: the tendency to blame ourselves when we shouldn't.

Burnout is not your fault

The most important thing to remember is that burnout is not your fault. The American Medical Association website has a detailed analysis of the drivers of burnout. As discussed earlier, only about 20 to 25% of those drivers are under your control. As a reminder, areas that are either not in your control or over which you have minimal control include factors like your work unit, your healthcare organization, and even state and national factors. Let's look at each of these in more detail.

Work unit factors include productivity expectations, team structure, and your workload, as well as your ability to get support from your staff and the use of allied health professionals to share the load. Supportive interactions with your superiors, peers, and staff can help recharge your energy, whereas a lack of support or a hostile or toxic environment in your work unit can be a major source of stress and drain your energy. Your ability to exert some control over the environment—including work hours and workload, call schedule and compensation—decreases your risk for burnout.

Important institutional or **organizational factors** include management and their expectations. Organizational culture is critical because it tends to flow from the top down. An organization's mission, vision, and values can have a positive impact if they align with yours. However, they can have a negative impact if senior leaders' actual behavior does not match their stated mission and values, or if they're not in line with *your* top values.

One of the most important organizational factors recently has been the selection of and implementation of electronic health records (EHR.) If the acquisition and implementation of EHR accounts for doctors and nurses' needs, it can be relatively painless. If, however, this selection and implementation process does not include feedback from the clinical users and improvement based on that feedback, it can become a focus for resentment and stress.

Finally, there are **national factors** of the healthcare system at large which are not in your control. This includes the structure of reimbursement systems, and whether they are federally or state funded or through private insurance networks. The level of reimbursement, documentation requirements, certifications, and restrictions can add to the administrative burden and stress on the physician or nurse that contribute to burnout.

Now that you understand that burnout is not your fault *nor* your failing, it's easier to see burnout as a symptom, not a disease. It is a sign that the healthcare system as it is now is failing. While this system does a fairly good job of taking care of its patients, and a *very* good job of taking care of its executives and investors, it falls short in caring for its doctors, nurses and other frontline healthcare providers. Dr. Drummond likens this situation to the "canary in a coal mine." For those who aren't familiar with this analogy: in the old days of coal mining, the greatest threat to the miners other than a cave-in was the accumulation of invisible odorless toxic gasses. Because canaries are very sensitive to those gasses, the miners would bring a canary in a cage down into the mine. When the canary stopped singing, the miners would know the toxic gas level was too high and they would get out right away. Using this analogy, burnout is a sign that the current healthcare system is toxic to providers.

Unfortunately, many "burnout prevention" programs—especially those designed by administrators—are focused on increasing physician resilience. That is the equivalent of building a stronger canary and ignoring the underlying toxic systemic problems. Fortunately, there are ways of improving the system that results in better outcomes for healthcare providers, patients and healthcare organizations as well. One is to utilize Lean Sigma management consistently and organization wide. I will discuss some of the other individual strategies in the chapter on teamwork.

Now that you know the causes of burnout, you're ready to learn how to protect yourself, your patients and your family from the damage caused by this symptom. In the next ten chapters, I will give you a series of actionable steps you can take to empower yourself and take back control of your life.

Key Points:

1. Burnout is characterized by mental and physical exhaustion, cynicism and loss of empathy and a loss of self-efficacy.

2. Burnout is very common among healthcare professionals and has profound personal and professional consequences.

3. There are 5 main causes of burnout: the practice of clinical medicine, your specific local work environment, our upbringing and academic training, our unconscious beliefs that

we have to be perfect and never ask for help, and the failure of leadership in our healthcare organizations and government.

4. Burnout is not your fault. It is not a personal failing. It is a symptom of the failure of healthcare systems and organizations to take care of the needs of frontline healthcare providers.

5. Only 20-25% of the causative factors of burnout are within your control; but that's enough to make a real difference in your life. In the following chapters of this book I will show you some simple steps to take to empower yourself and make that difference.

References:

https://www.mywellbeingindex.org/

https://nam.edu/gender-based-differences-in-burnout-issues-faced-by-women-physicians/

https://www.aafp.org/fpm/2015/0900/p42.html

Chapter 2

GET A COACH

You might be wondering: why do I need a coach? After all, you're not a professional athlete. You're a doctor, or a nurse, or a healthcare manager, or executive. You may wonder about the value of coaching, and what can you get from it – and might also be thinking, "Isn't there some way I can straighten out my life *without* a coach?"

I know it sounds a little bit self-serving, since I *am* a coach, so I'm not going to recommend you simply take my word for it. This chapter provides evidence and anecdotes on exactly what coaching can do for you and why you should have a coach. Of course, coaching has been used in sports for as long as athletic history has been recorded. In today's world, no professional, college athlete, high school, or even grade school athletes would consider trying to achieve superior performance without a coach.

So, what does an athletic coach do? Well, we know he or she does not actually play the game, although they may have played it in the past. Rather, a coach's skill lies in recognizing the athletes' untapped abilities and helping them reach peak performance. Coaches are able to observe the athlete in action from an objective point of view and see how that athlete can fine-tune their skills to achieve maximum performance. Although general skills can be taught, coaching is essentially a one-on-one interaction (unless involved in a team sport). That's because every player or athlete has a different set of skills and strengths, and a different level of potential. It's up to the coach to help the athlete to build on their existing strengths and build new ones from areas of weakness.

But coaching in athletics is not all about the physical game. This process is explained beautifully in Tim Galway's book *The Inner Game of Tennis*. Galway explains that there is both an inner game and an outer game taking place with all sports. The outer game is what you see played out on the court or in the field; but the inner game is played out in the athlete's mind. Therefore, coaching has to cover both areas. Sometimes, even professional athletes' biggest obstacles are in the inner game—through self-doubt, negative self-talk, or unproductive thoughts. It is only when the inner game and outer game are fully in alignment that the athlete enters "the zone" and can perform at his or her highest level.

The effectiveness of athletic coaching is fairly easily quantified—either in points or scores or money made. The effectiveness of personal or life coaching is not as easily quantified. However, we can measure this by the client's success in reaching their personal goals, improving their relationships and experiencing general feelings of optimism and well-being.

Coaching entered the business arena around 1985-1990 with executive coaching. Most often, coaches are called either to assist executives who are moving up in the organization and need to polish their managerial skills. Less often, coaches are called when managers or executives are felt to be underperforming. Coaching is also used extensively in sales to help increase motivation and productivity. As with athletic coaching, the benefits of business coaching can be semi-quantified in terms of dollar amounts, amounts of increased productivity or increased sales. Using these metrics, research into the cost and benefits of business coaching has yielded a return on investment of between 300% and 500%. Wouldn't you like to get that kind of return on some of your other investments? And those numbers don't even reflect other benefits, such as quality of life and employee engagement.

So, why would a healthcare professional need coaching? The economic advantages are clear for a healthcare organization or medical group. If coaching can help prevent or reduce burnout among doctors and nurses, there's direct correlation with turnover. And as I mentioned before, the cost of replacing a primary care physician—an expense that includes lost productivity, recruitment, and training—approaches $900,000. For a nurse, that number is approximately $200,000. A recent article in Annals of Internal Medicine put the overall cost of physician burnout to the medical system at $4.6 billion annually! And that doesn't include the cost of medical errors and malpractice suits.

The personal advantages are more difficult to quantify, but just as important. We can measure these using metrics such as quality of life scales or, more recently, previously mentioned burnout indicators like the Maslach Inventory or the Well-Being Index. These measurements are only semi-quantitative, since all of them are based on self-reporting. Nevertheless, research to date demonstrates significant improvement in quality of life and goal attainment on an individual level through coaching.

These benefits have been repeatedly demonstrated in the coaching literature as shown by the figure below. This graph, which is a synopsis of several studies on life coaching, shows that attainment of personal and professional goals is markedly improved in people undergoing coaching versus those that try on their own

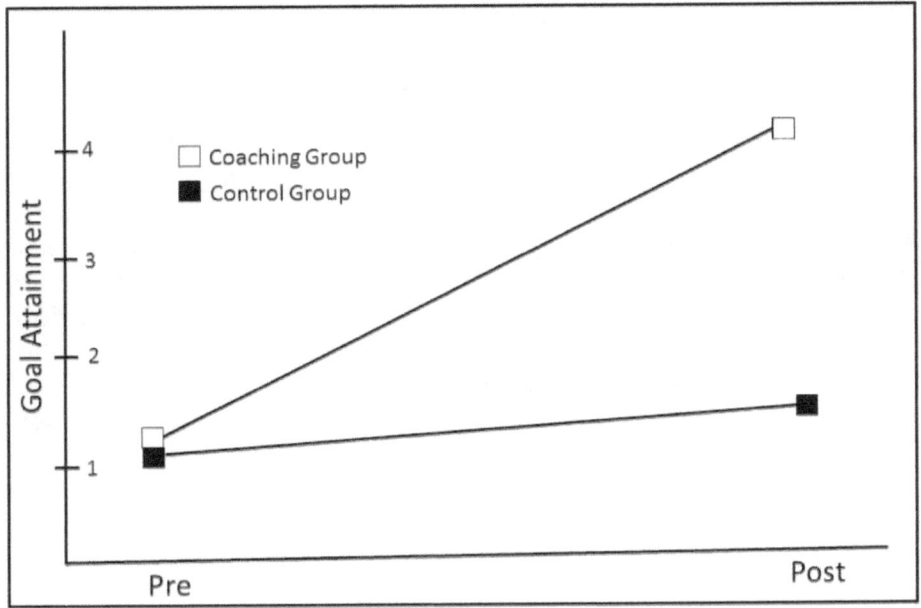

What is the difference between coaching and therapy?

Coaching is different from therapy, consulting, and mentoring in several important ways. Although many coaches come from a psychology or therapy background, not all do. Coaching is a supplement to, not a substitute for therapy if you already have a psychiatric diagnosis, are on psychoactive medications, are severely depressed, or having thoughts of harming yourself or others. If these conditions are present, it's very important to **maintain your therapy treatment plan and medications** and to inform your therapist that you're also undergoing a coaching process.

Having said that, there are some advantages of coaching that are absent from therapy. Coaches spend less time trying to figure out how you got where you are, and more time helping you figure out where you want to go and how to get there. In a coaching relationship, the coach and client work together in a cooperative arrangement that helps the client to make and achieve goals. The coach may act as a sounding board and an accountability partner, but the client does the actual change work and is responsible for their own results. Another significant advantage of coaching, assuming that therapy is not indicated, is that coaches are not required to report to the medical board.

It's also important to remember that a coach is not a **consultant or mentor**. A consultant uses their expertise and experience to help identify problems and propose solutions. A **mentor**, on the other hand, is someone who uses the benefit of their experience to share what they have learned. He or she may help the mentee move in their desired direction by providing encouragement, and sometimes by using their own reputation and influence to help the mentee. Both consultants and mentors are assumed to be the experts in their field. A coach, on the other hand, assumes that you are the expert in your own life, and with guidance will come up with your own best solutions.

The AMA recognizes the value of coaching

In 2019 the AMA recognized the value of coaching by approving specific CPT codes for coaches certified by the National Board for Health and Wellness Coaches, a subsidiary of the National Board of Medical Examiners (the same board that certifies doctors.) Current Procedural Terminology (**CPT**) is a medical code set that is used to report medical, surgical, and diagnostic procedures and services to entities such as physicians, health insurance companies and accreditation organizations. The AMA defines a coach as a non-physician health care professional certified by NBHWC or NCHEC. The approved Health and Well-Being Coaching Category III CPT® codes will be in effect for five years but are renewable. These temporary codes are intended to support the wide utilization and data collection, with and without reimbursement, required for AMA approval of Category 1 codes. Reimbursement by payors of Category III codes is optional starting January 1, 2020, but payors typically wait until codes have Category I approval to begin reimbursement.

About the National Board for Health & Wellness Coaching (NBHWC)

NBHWC and the National Board of Medical Examiners (NBME) launched national standards and board certification for health and wellness coaches in 2017. There are currently 2,300+ National Board-Certified Health & Wellness Coaches (NBC-HWC), including me, practicing across healthcare, employee wellness programs, and in the private and public sectors. For more information visit https://nbhwc.org.

How do you define the coaching relationship?

The following is the definition from the **International Coaching Federation:**

"Coaching is partnering with clients in a thought-provoking and creative process that inspires them to maximize their potential, their personal and professional potential."

The next definition is from the **Association for Coaching:**

"Coaching is a collaborative, solution-focus, results-oriented, and systematic process in which the coach facilitates the enhancement of work performance, life experience, self-directed learning, and personal growth of the coachee."

I personally like the way that author and coach Kate Burton sums up the definition of coaching in her book *Coaching for Dummies:*

"Whatever your definition, coaching is a relationship that brings out the very best in both client and coach. During coaching, a special conversation takes place that's completely focused on the client's needs in a way that empowers him to dream bigger dreams, increase his performance, articulate what he wants, and work out how to get what he most desires."

How do you know if you're ready for coaching?

Use the set of questions in the box below to see if you're at a point where you should consider hiring a coach. If you can't answer yes to these questions, or if you have other questions, then you should have a conversation with a coach before engaging their services. The good news is that most coaches will provide a free exploratory conversation or a phone call where they'll help answer your questions.

Try This:

If you can agree with the 8 statements below, you are ready to be coached:

1. I will keep appointments with myself to work on my coaching homework

2. There is something I want to work on or achieve which I will focus on in my coaching.

3. I am willing to stop or change behaviors that are interfering with my progress.

4. I am willing to try new approaches to help me achieve my goals.

5. Coaching is an appropriate approach to help me accomplish my goals, as opposed to therapy for an emotional issue, consulting for specific problem solving, or specific teaching.

6. I will take regular actions to help achieve my coaching goals even if I don't see immediate results.

7. I will be open with my coach about what I like or don't like about how the coaching is going.

8. I will work collaboratively with my coach to design goals and action steps to move forward.

Usually before you proceed with a coaching engagement, there is a coaching contract which specifies both the coach's and the client's obligations in the relationship, as well as the type and timing of scheduled meetings and financial arrangements.

Using NLP and coaching together

A small minority of coaches, including me, are additionally trained in integrative neurolinguistic coaching. This is a combination of positive psychology coaching and neurolinguistic programming. Neurolinguistic programming (NLP) is a psychological approach to behavioral change using the structure of language as a tool to intentionally re-structure thought patterns and beliefs in order to achieve the client's goals. It was developed in the 1970's as part of the "humanistic psychology" movement, the precursor to today's positive psychology. This combination of approaches, in my experience, may allow the client to make more rapid progress, especially if he or she is being held back by inner conflicts, limiting beliefs, or unresolved emotions from the past.

Author and coach Kate Burton describes the value of combining NLP and coaching in her book *Coaching with NLP for Dummies* as follows:

"An NLP client may experience a dramatic breakthrough at a single intensive session while coaching tends to have it its ups and downs over a period of sessions. Indeed, an individual coaching session may not seem important at the time, yet it contributes to some deeper understanding in the longer term. Coaching and NLP take different routes to achieve the same end result, to leave the clients in a better place physically, emotionally, mentally, or spiritually than when they started. Both disciplines address challenges of self-awareness and relationships with others. Bring NLP and coaching together, and you have a winning combination to find the unconscious brilliance in each human being."

Finally, there's the question of whether you should do group or individual coaching. Some advantages of group coaching are that it is a more economical way than individual coaching to "test drive" the coaching process. In addition, working in a group gives you an instant peer support structure. Group coaching works well in an online format where the clients in the group can interact with the coach and with each other in real time. I used this format in my medical student group coaching.

There are also many advantages to individual coaching, including receiving one-on-one attention from your coach and maintaining complete confidentiality. There is an opportunity to explore specific areas of life at a deeper level. In addition, there are some specific techniques or tools of coaching such as NLP that are best done one-on-one. Working with a coach one-on-one, a client often makes rapid progress and can work on new situations as they arise. Many of my clients are so motivated by the changes in one area of life that they extend the original coaching engagement to work on new goals or other areas of life.

Key Points:

1. Get a coach. Interview a couple of coaches to find one that you feel Is right for you. Most coaches offer a free discovery session where you can share your goals and get your questions answered.

2. Make sure you're ready to be coached and make the time and financial commitment for at least 3-6 months to see if you're getting the results you want.

3. Commit to doing the work in and in-between coaching sessions. Like most activities, you get out what you put in.

References:

Auerbach, J, The Well-Being Coaching Workbook, Executive College Press, Pismo Beach, CA 2014

Burton, Kate. Coaching with NLP For Dummies. Wiley. Kindle Edition

Chapter 3

PRACTICE MINDFULNESS

What if I told you that there was a simple five-minute procedure that can decrease stress, increase your self-confidence, enhance your focus and concentration, help you become more calm and centered, improve your communication skills, *and* build better relationships? I'm guessing that's something that would interest you—and those are some of the direct benefits of practicing **mindfulness.**

The practice of mindfulness has been studied scientifically for the last 50 years. It has been shown to decrease stress, increase recovery from physical or mental illness, and to reduce the incidence of work-related burnout. In just 5 or 10 minutes a day, you can increase your focus and concentration in a way that will save you hours at work. You can also cultivate a state of mind that allows you to be truly present for your family or children, or other people who are important in your life

I'll explain another form of mindfulness practice that you can do in 30 seconds or less to eliminate negative thoughts and emotions at any time during the day, and to reset your emotional thermostat whenever you need to. In the following chapters, I will also be talking about the importance of **boundary rituals.** These show how we can use mindfulness practice to clearly separate our workday from our home life, or separate different parts of our workday or different tasks in a way that allows us to effortlessly and easily be more productive.

What is mindfulness?

Mindfulness is simply a way of paying attention by observing whatever is happening in the present moment, without judgment. The first written explanation of a kind of mindfulness known as breath meditation is from approximately 500 BCE by the Buddha, Siddhartha Gautama. He describes at the beginning that mindfulness of the breath, "when developed and repeatedly practiced, is of great benefit and ultimately can lead to clear vision and enlightenment." He then goes on to describe the exact method of practicing breath meditation, which I will share with you in this chapter. In the Buddhist tradition, the practice of mindfulness is thought to develop focus and concentration, which leads to deep insights and the experience of Nirvana or enlightenment. It's important to keep in mind that although the practice of mindfulness was first described within a religious or philosophical context, mindfulness itself is a human characteristic. It is totally separate from the practice of a given religion, philosophy or spirituality.

Of course, the attainment of enlightenment often takes many years of mindfulness practice, and most of us don't have the luxury of time and leisure to practice for hours a day, years on end. Interestingly, enlightenment is sometimes translated as "liberation." "Liberation from what?" You may wonder. It is liberation from what I call the "big five" limiting emotions: anger, sadness, fear, hurt, and guilt. Freeing yourself of those negative emotions may only require five to ten minutes of mindfulness practice a day on a regular basis. Think about how much better your life would be without the big five standing in the way of your goals, your relationships, and your ability to enjoy life.

Before I share the instructions for mindfulness meditation, I would like to share with you my own odyssey on the road to liberation so you can see how anyone, including you, can grow spiritually. Of course your journey need not be so long. Now, through the power of the internet, world renowned spiritual teachers (even those no longer with us) are available at your fingertips. You don't need to travel to an Indian ashram or even physically go to a retreat, (although I recommend that you try it because a retreat can accelerate your practice; sharing meditation in a room with other people multiplies the level of mindfulness.) So, let your fingers do the travelling and explore the world of mindfulness online.

My mindfulness journey

For many years, I was a spiritual seeker. Like many other baby boomers, I was a big fan of the Beatles' music. In the 1970s, the Beatles became devotees of a spiritual teacher named Maharishi Mahesh Yogi. The change in their attitude and music under his direction impressed me enough that I wanted to learn that form of meditation—a mantra meditation known as Transcendental Meditation (TM.) So I sought out my local TM group and paid the required fee to get my "secret" mantra, which was a word I was to repeat silently to myself as an object of meditation. While I found TM to be a useful practice for myself, eventually I was turned off by the cult-like characteristics of the organization and their emphasis on material wealth. Somehow, I did not see the 12 Rolls Royces that the Maharishi owned as the appropriate vehicles for enlightenment.

After that, for a period of time, I followed Ram Dass—former Harvard professor Richard Alpert and the author of the wonderful little book entitled *Be Here Now*. I then discovered the teachings of a modest Vietnamese Zen Buddhist monk named Thich Nhat Hanh, who was coming to the United States to promote peace in Vietnam and to make the practice of mindfulness easily accessible to westerners. His anti-war activism led to his nomination for the Nobel Peace Prize by Martin Luther King in 1967. In the 1980s, Hanh began giving mindfulness retreats in the United States—first in Upstate New York and later in California, many of which I attended. He was my main spiritual teacher from that time until 2014, when he suffered a stroke and could no longer teach.

Another person who was greatly influenced by the teachings of Thich Nhat Hanh was Dr. Jon Kabat-Zinn at the University of Massachusetts Medical Center. In 1979, Dr. Kabat-Zinn founded the Stress Reduction Clinic at UMass Medical School. Here, he adapted the Buddhist teachings on mindfulness to help patients cope with the stress, pain, and illnesses they suffered. Since that time, his eight-week structured course called Mindfulness Based Stress Reduction or MBSR has been extensively studied. It is now an accepted part of not only treatment of patients with chronic illnesses, but also in supporting the medical professionals who care for those patients. Thousands of published studies have established MBSR as an adjunct to medical treatment that reduces the suffering caused by pain and anxiety, improves healing and brain function, and even improves immune system functioning. It has also been shown to decrease the rate of burnout among nurses, doctors, and other health professionals and to help those suffering from burnout to recover more quickly.

Dr. Kabat-Zinn's work took the practice of mindfulness from a religious framework and firmly established it within the scientific world. Although he is now retired, I had the pleasure of attending several weeklong mindfulness retreats for health care practitioners that he led. In those retreats I found like-minded practitioners determined to integrate mindfulness into their practices. They were the inspiring pioneers in what was called "mind-body medicine." Today we recognize that there really is no separation of the mind and body, as the sciences of psychoneuroimmunology (the study of relationships between the mind, neurologic and immune systems) and epigenetics (the study of how experiences affect the expression of human genes) have proven, and we have moved into the era of **integrative medicine**.

How do you practice mindfulness?

Simply put, mindfulness is an open state of mind where one observes what arises in the thoughts and in the five senses in the present moment without any filtering or judgment. Although mindfulness can be practiced at any moment and in any activity, people most commonly start with a "formal" mindfulness practice. This involves sitting still in a quiet place and paying attention to any sensory or thought object that occurs in the present moment, like breathing or looking at a candle flame, or repeating a word (mantra). This formal practice is called meditation and makes it easy to recognize anything that arises in consciousness that is *not* the object of meditation (like random thoughts, emotions, or physical sensations.)

Most people find it helpful at the beginning to have some kind of guidance while learning to meditate. The simplest form of guidance is a recording which can guide you through the process of achieving and maintaining mindfulness. Many recordings can be downloaded from mindfulness websites, YouTube, or even my own website:

https://www.gideonstrichmd.com/download-the-free-mindfulness-practice-mp3/

There are also many apps that you can use on your cell phone or tablet that guide you in mindfulness. You can find these by searching for mindfulness or meditation in your app store. My personal favorite is an app called "Headspace", which is the one that I recommend to my clients. There is a monthly subscription fee, although the first ten days are free if you want to give it a test drive. I like this particular app best because it not only guides you in the practice of meditation as you become more advanced, it also helps you deal with the obstacles that inevitably arise as you practice. such as self-doubt, loss of focus, or just a busy "monkey mind" on some days.

The basic instructions for mindfulness meditation using the breath are as follows:

First, sit in a comfortable, stable position with the spine straight but relaxed. You can sit on a meditation cushion in lotus (cross-legged) position, or kneel while sitting on a cushion or bench, or simply sit upright in a chair. If you sit in a chair, it is helpful to put a small cushion underneath your buttocks to allow your spine to be upright without being supported by the chair back. Putting your feet flat on the floor gives an additional sense of stability. Then either close the eyes or lower your gaze and allow your eyes to defocus.

Then, just bring your attention to the physical sensations associated with breathing. You may notice the flow of air in the nose or in the throat, or the rising and falling sensation of chest and abdomen. If you have a hard time noticing these sensations, simply gently place a hand on your abdomen and notice how it rises and falls naturally with the breath.

Just allow the breath to occur at its natural pace. Do not make any attempt to change it in any way. Allow yourself to focus gently on the sensations of breathing in a nonjudgmental manner. There is no "right" way to breathe. Every breath is exactly as valuable as any other, whether it is short or long, shallow or deep, fast or slow. You will probably notice after a very short period of time that your mind wanders off in thought. When you notice that your mind has wandered off, simply gently bring it back to the awareness of breathing. It is this process of recognizing when the mind has wandered and bringing it back to the breath that is the essence of mindfulness practice. Although your thoughts may quiet somewhat, they will always be present and there is no need to try to suppress them (or beat yourself up for letting your mind "wander".) When you become aware of thoughts, simply return your awareness to the physical sensation of breathing.

Some people find it helpful at the beginning to count the breaths silently, counting one with the in breath, two with the out breath, three with the next in breath, four with the next out breath, all the way up to 10, and then beginning again at one. If your mind wanders before you get to 10, simply pick up where you left off or begin again at one. It doesn't really matter. Some days you will never get to 10 before your mind wanders, but just be patient and begin again each time the same way. You can time your meditation session using a guided meditation or one of the many meditation timing apps available such as "Insight Timer" or "Mind Bell."

Mindfulness is considered a "practice" because it gradually improves over time with regular practice. Just like developing a muscle, you don't develop mindfulness with a single session. Rather, the recommendation is to practice 10 to 20 minutes twice a day, although even five minutes once a day will make a noticeable improvement in your life.

How to Practice Mindful Breathing

1. Sit in a comfortable stable position with a straight spine. You can sit on a meditation cushion or a straight back chair with your feet flat on the floor.

2. Most people practice with eyes closed, but you can keep your eyes open and your gaze downcast and defocused.

3. Bring your attention to the physical sensations of breathing. You may notice coolness in the nose, or movement of air in the throat or the rise and fall of the chest or abdomen.

4. Don't focus too hard; just be gently aware. There is no right or wrong way to breath. Just allow your breath to come and go in its own natural rhythm.

5. When you notice that your attention has drifted away from the breath to some thoughts or feelings, just let go of those thoughts and gently bring your attention back to the breath.

6. It is this process of gently redirecting your attention back to the physical sensations of breathing over and over again that is the essence of training the mind and developing mindfulness.

7. Training the mind is like training your muscles. It works best if you practice every day even if it's only for 5-10 minutes.

8. Turn it into a habit by making time for mindful breathing in between two habits you already do every day at about the same time.

Another form of mindfulness practice that I use based on Thich Nhat Hanh's teachings is what I call the 30 second meditation, or the **single breath meditation.** This process takes less than 30 seconds and can be practiced multiple times during the day. It does not require any special place, position or even eye closure. It is a way of releasing negative energy and calming the mind. It can also be used as a **boundary ritual** – for example, in between home and work, or work and home, or even in between patient encounters. If you don't see patients, you can even practice this whenever you answer the phone. Thich Nhat Hanh referred to this as "telephone meditation," and this is how you do it:

First, either close your eyes or simply defocus the gaze. Take a slow deep breath into the abdomen, gathering up any excess or any negative energy that you're aware of, or *anything* that you're aware of that doesn't serve you at this moment. As you allow your breath to escape, feel as though you could breathe all this negative energy into the ground through the bottom of your feet. Then pause at the bottom of the out-breath for three or four seconds, just noticing the silence and the space that you feel in that moment. Then take in a normal breath, open your eyes and go back to your business while trying to maintain that mindful awareness. The 30-second meditation works well to help you set boundaries between different personal and professional interactions, and helps you be fully present for patients and your family (which we'll talk more about in Chapter 11.)

Bringing mindfulness into everyday life

If you practice mindfulness on a regular basis—especially sitting mindfulness meditation for five to ten minutes a day— you will find that gradually, mindfulness will extend beyond the sitting period into your everyday life. You become increasingly aware of how your thoughts and emotions affect your behavior. That recognition allows you to recognize that **you are not your thoughts and emotions.** Thoughts and feelings simply arise and fade away naturally. There is no need to push them away, nor is there any need to hold onto them. This, then, is the beginning of your liberation from the tyranny of thoughts and of emotions, and the beginning of your freedom to make intelligent choices in your life on a day to day and moment to moment basis. This is how you reclaim control over the results in your life. That is called **empowerment.**

Try this:

The ten-day mindfulness challenge:

1. Download a mindfulness meditation app (like Headspace) and practice every morning for 5 minutes. Set aside the time and space to do this even if you have to get up 5 minutes earlier. Make it a priority.

2. Practice the single breath meditation in the car before entering the workplace and again just before entering your home after work. Say to yourself, "With this breath I let go of anything that doesn't need to be here right now, and I come all the way back to the present moment."

3. Repeat #2 several times during the day and associate it with another action you know you will be taking during the day, like just before you enter a patient room or just before you answer the phone. Make it a habit.

4. Make a note of how this practice affects your mood, your calmness, and your ability to be truly present for your patients and your family.

Key Points:

1. Cultivating mindfulness is the foundation of reducing stress and burnout, increasing mental focus and concentration, and improving communication and relationships. That is why it is the first skill I practice with my coaching clients.

2. Simple breath meditation requires no special place or position, and is completely free of religion, belief, age or gender. It is a simple human ability.

3. The regular practice of mindfulness liberates you from the "big five" limiting emotions of anger, sadness, fear, hurt and guilt. It gives you more freedom in how you live your life and it results in personal empowerment.

4. You can use the single breath meditation as a boundary ritual between home and work and between work and home, or at any time during the day you feel stressed.

Chapter 4

KEEP A JOURNAL

O nce you've discovered the amazing power of developing mindfulness and have established a mindfulness practice every morning for five to 10 minutes, you can introduce another simple habit that can change your entire life: journaling or keeping a journal. Many people associate the word *journaling* with the notion of teenage girls' diaries or the intellectuals of the 19th century. But that view of writing a journal is entirely outmoded, and there is a lot of research supporting the value of journaling nowadays.

One of the benefits of journaling supported by scientific evidence is that it's shown to increase your mindfulness in *all* areas of life. In this way, journaling builds on the foundation that you've already developed through your mindfulness practice. Writing about your feelings and experiences can increase your emotional intelligence, a characteristic which is associated with both improved executive abilities at work and enhanced overall communication and quality of relationships. We will explore this area in Chapter 9 in the section on rapport and communication.

Journaling has been shown to increase your creativity and your vocabulary range; over time, it also makes you more articulate and more interesting. It's been shown to reduce stress, especially when combined with mindfulness. It may improve your mood and has been proven in clinical trials to help relieve symptoms of depression.

Task-oriented journaling helps you achieve your goals and keep track of your progress on your action steps. This type of journaling is critical in setting and accomplishing your goals and in helping maintain your accountability to yourself. Your coach will assist you in this process. Journaling allows you to build self-confidence; scientific studies have even shown that it can improve immune function and stimulate healing, which we'll discuss more in this next section.

The emotional advantage of journaling

Social psychologist Dr. James Pennebaker of the University of Texas, Austin reviewed a large number of studies on the positive effects of journaling and summarized them in a 1999 article in the *Journal of Clinical Psychology*. Here are some highlights from that article.

"The act of constructing stories is a natural human process that helps individuals understand their experiences and themselves." Since the beginning of human language, people have used stories to understand themselves and their place in the world. Story telling is the most effective and widespread way that we communicate our ideas and beliefs. Tribes, communities and countries are drawn together through shared narratives.

"Extensive research has revealed that when people put their emotional upheavals into words, their physical and mental health improves markedly." In a study with college students, Pennebaker found that just writing about their deepest thoughts and feeling resulted in improvement of their physical and mental health and even improved their grades!

In his article, Dr. Pennebaker reviewed results of previous journaling research, extending back over a decade. He summarizes articles that have found that benefits of journaling occur across widely differing populations, ranging from college students to maximum security prisoners, from chronic pain sufferers to crime victims. The positive effects have been found in all social classes and major racial and ethnic groups, both in United States and abroad. In short – journaling helps almost anyone you can imagine.

Journaling also affects our health and immune systems positively. Not only can we infer this information from decreased physician visits and medication use we see in those who take the time to journal; we can also see it measured objectively in the laboratory by changes in T-cell function and antibody response. The effect of journaling on both short- and long-term mood effects are quite interesting. Although people writing about traumatic events tended to feel more unhappy and distressed in the hours immediately following the writing, two weeks later those people reported being happier than members of groups who did not do any journaling.

According to Pennebaker, "The emotional state after writing depends on how participants are feeling prior to writing: The better they feel before writing, the worse they feel afterwards and vice versa." But a day later, both groups feel better than before. Pennebaker summarizes the research as follows, "Writing about important personal experiences in an emotional way, for as little as 15 minutes over the course of three days, brings about improvement in mental and physical health." This finding has been replicated across age, gender, culture, social class and personality type.

How to begin journaling

First, decide on a medium for recording your thoughts and feelings. Some studies have shown that handwriting your journal is more effective than typing or speaking and integrates more areas of brain function. There are also many apps available online and on portable devices that make journaling much more convenient. Some people use general note taking apps such as Evernote, Trello or Microsoft One Note. There are many specific journaling apps. Some of the popular ones include Dalio, Diario and Journey. There are literally hundreds more in your app store. I have developed a journaling app specific to my type of mindfulness-based coaching that not only makes journaling easy but gives my clients quantitative feedback on their progress over time.

Regardless of the medium, what's important is to get something down in written format – so choose something you're likely to use. Ideally, you should write once a day. I recommend that my clients write in the evening while the memories of the day's events are fresh. It is important to set aside a private time—at least five to ten minutes—when you know you won't be interrupted.

Your journal can be structured or unstructured, depending on what you're looking to get out of the journaling process. Unstructured or stream of thought journaling is better for expressing thoughts and feelings and dealing with emotional trauma. However, a more structured approach may be helpful for goal setting, prioritizing and organizing your day,. One such approach is the "bullet journal", described by Ryder Carol in his book, *The Bullet Journal Method*. This method uses separate pages for daily, weekly and monthly goals with specific symbols to denote tasks to do, appointments, people to contact, and priorities. You can even incorporate introspective notes on the day's events and doodles or artwork. Carol sees this method as an analog antidote to digital overload, a way to sort out what's really important to you and intentionally focus on that. As he puts it, "The Bullet Journal method will help you accomplish more by working on less. It helps you identify and focus on what is meaningful by stripping away what is meaningless."

Regardless of whether you're using an unstructured or structured journal, the most important thing is to make journaling a consistent habit. Taking only five minutes a day to journal is perfectly acceptable as long as it's five minutes *every day*. You can make your journaling process part of a boundary ritual so that it serves two purposes., a quiet time for introspection and integrating the day's events, and a boundary between that day and the beginning of the next day. We'll go into more detail on the importance of habits and boundary rituals in a later chapter. If you are writing about an emotional or traumatic event, you don't have to recall all the details or relive the trauma. You can simply write about whatever you're feeling in the present moment at whatever level of detail you find comfortable. Since the goal is to form a habit you'll want to repeat, you don't want to engage in any behavior you might start to dread or avoid.

A good set of guidelines on how to journal effectively can be found on the website for The Center for Journal Therapy. They use the acronym **WRITE**, which is explained in detail below.

The WRITE Process

W: What should you write about? You can write about events that are occurring in your life or any thoughts and feelings about past events or future goals and desires.

R: Reflect for a few moments before you start writing. This might be a perfect time to do the single-breath or 30-second meditation to bring yourself into mindfulness in the present moment.

I: Investigate what you are currently thinking and feeling and just start to put those thoughts and feelings into writing without too much analysis or editing. It helps if you begin sentences with I statements like I feel, I think, I want, and focus on the present moment by using words like right now or today.

T: Time yourself so that you write for a set period of time, whether it's 5 minutes or 10 minutes. Make a note of your start time and expected end time and set a timer when you begin. When the timer goes off, simply stop writing wherever you are.

E: Exiting the writing session. Take a few moments to reread what you've written and reflect on it. Take another single-breath meditation. Summarize your session and its takeaways in one or two sentences. And then if there are any specific actions that you wish to take in the next day, make a note of those as well.

Make it a point to find a time to write, even if it's only for five minutes per day. Try to write for the same amount of time each day and at the same time. It may be helpful to use habit stacking; that is, to use a habit that you have already established to remind you to begin the habit of journaling. You can put that habit stack into words, such as "Every evening after I finish dinner and before I watch TV, I will take five minutes to journal my thoughts and feelings." That way, the habit of journaling is stacked between two habits you've already established: eating dinner and watching TV. After doing this for a couple of weeks, it will become a new habit, and you will start to see some of the benefits of journaling.

Journaling helps you manage stress and decrease anxiety. The practice of journaling has been shown not only to strengthen the immune system, but also to decrease blood pressure and help you sleep better. Journaling helps decrease anxiety by making us more mindful of our negative self-talk, which in turn helps us take a more balanced view of our lives. We can note certain experiences that have caused us stress or anxiety and find out what triggers those feelings. By intentionally writing about positive events in our day, journaling can make us more aware of our strengths and inner resources and gives us a more balanced view of ourselves.

If you're writing about a specific traumatic event or if you're suffering from an eating disorder or other psychological condition, journaling can be a great *adjunct* to psychotherapy. It allows you to make progress in between sessions by processing the thoughts and emotions associated with stressful events and noticing how dysfunctional behaviors result from specific triggers. Eventually, noticing the less helpful way we react to these things can help us understand how to respond differently. One of the most traumatic events is the loss of someone close to us, and journaling about that loss can help us process the emotions and to rebound more quickly from grief.

Journaling can help manage depression and decrease its effects by reducing brooding and rumination, which are two factors that contribute to depression. Gratitude journaling has been shown specifically to improve mood and decrease symptoms of depression; we will talk about that specifically in the chapter on positivity and happiness.

Try this:

1. Find a time at the end of the day when you can be alone in a private place to journal.

2. Make it the same time every day and for the same amount of time, between 5 and 10 minutes. Use habit stacking as described above.

3. Decide on a medium for journaling. It can be a journaling app or a notebook and pen.

4. Journal about any event that occurred during the day, even a seemingly insignificant event.

   a. Start with a single breath meditation (see chapter 3) to center yourself and create a boundary around your journaling time.

   b. Set a timer for the amount of time you have decided on.

   c. Begin writing and keep writing until the timer goes off.

   d. Stop and read what you have written and briefly reflect on it.

   e. Do another single breath meditation to finish the session

5. Do the above steps every day for two weeks until it becomes a habit.

6. Then take some time and reflect how it has affected your feelings and your outlook on life.

Now that you've discovered how simple it is to begin and maintain a journaling practice—and the many benefits that can come as a result of writing down your thoughts and feelings even for five minutes a day—give it a try yourself. Commit to taking and completing the 14-day challenge above and see how much of difference it makes.

In the next chapter, we will talk specifically about happiness and why most people are looking for happiness in the wrong places. We will build on what you learned in this chapter by discussing how to use journaling as one of the roads to lasting happiness in your life and to better, more fulfilling relationships.

Key Points:

1. Along with a regular mindfulness practice, a regular journaling habit is the single most useful and transformative activity you can do.

2. Scientific research shows that journaling can improve your communication skills and your overall health, and reduce the negative effects of stress, anxiety and depression.

3. Like mindfulness practice, journaling has its most powerful effect if you do it every day for a set period of time (5-10 minutes) at about the same time of day. Use habit stacking to help you remember to do it.

References:

https://journaltherapy.com

Pennebaker J and Seagal J. Forming a Story: The Health Benefits of Narrative. J Clin Psychol 55: 1243-1254, 1999.

Carroll R. The Bullet Journal Method: Track the Past, Order the Present, Design the Future. Kindle Edition. Penguin Group. 2018

CULTIVATE POSITIVITY

Most people will tell you that being happy is one of the main goals in their lives. However, most people have a hard time describing what happiness is. In this chapter we will be exploring what happiness is and how you can intentionally cultivate happiness in your life.

What is happiness?

Many research psychologists use the term happiness interchangeably with "subjective wellbeing," which they measure by simply asking people to report how satisfied they feel with their own lives, and how much positive and negative emotion they're experiencing at the time. One researcher, psychologist Sonja Lyubomirsky, describes happiness as "the experience of joy, contentment, or positive wellbeing combined with a sense that one's life is good and meaningful and worthwhile." The following is a quote on happiness from the Greater Good website: "Most of us probably don't believe we need a formal definition of happiness. We know it when we feel it and we often use the term to describe a range of positive emotions, including joy, pride, contentment, and gratitude." *How would you describe what happiness is to you?*

The pursuit of happiness- The happiness trap

The idea of trying to pursue happiness is deeply embedded in western culture. In the United States, it is even enshrined in the most American of documents, the Declaration of Independence, which states that all men are entitled to "life, liberty, and the pursuit of happiness." Ironically, positive psychology research shows that the more value you place on your own happiness, the more likely you are to feel lonely. In an article by psychologist Robert Baumeister in *Journal of Positive Psychology*, he states that, "Happiness without meaning characterizes a relatively shallow, self-absorbed, or even selfish life."

One of the big problems with pursuing happiness is that most people either don't know where to look for it, or they look for it in the wrong place. One common question is, "Can money buy happiness?" The answer is both yes and no. Research has shown that increasing income up to a subsistence level that affords food, housing, and health security, *does* indeed correlate with increasing happiness. Depending upon the area of the country in which you live, the effects of increasing income on happiness taper off at between 75,000 and 100,00 dollars per year. After this point is reached, increasing income does *not* correlate with increasing happiness. It may in fact result in *decreased* happiness, because people expect their increased income to equal increased happiness—and that is not always the case.

So, where should we look for happiness? A 2011 article from the *Harvard Business Review* states that, "Of all the events that engage people at work, the single most important by far is simply making progress in meaningful work." So maybe we should be seeking not happiness itself, but a life of meaning. Interestingly, meaning in one's life is something that can be found even under the most arduous and horrific circumstances. In his 1946 book, psychiatrist Viktor Frankl chronicled his experiences as a prisoner in a Nazi concentration camp during World War II. Frankl concluded that happiness, or at least meaning, involved identifying a purpose in your life to feel positively about, and then vividly imagining the outcome. One of the lessons to be learned is that the process of making meaning in one's life is incremental, and even very small wins generate meaningful progress. I have found this to be true with many of my coaching clients. For example, even a minor improvement in their relationships may effect a positive change in their career trajectory and vice versa.

One of the most prolific researchers in the field of positive psychology, Dr. Barbara Fredrickson, doesn't even use the word happiness. In her 2009 book *Positivity*, she describes 10 forms of positivity, including joy, gratitude, serenity, interest, hope, pride, amusement, inspiration, awe, and love. She has proposed a "broaden and build model of positivity." Interestingly, this model is based on the development of mindfulness. According to Dr. Fredrickson, the state of mindfulness results in broadening of one's attention beyond the individual self, which leads to a more positive reappraisal of your condition, which then leads to more positive emotions and decreased stress. This decreased stress then prompts an increased state of mindfulness, further attentional broadening, and additional positive feelings in a continuing upward spiral of flourishing. An opposite downward spiral of psychopathology occurs when stress results in narrowing of attention and loss of mindfulness. This process results in increased negative emotions and a feeling of threat, which then leads to further narrowing of attention to the self, more negative emotions and increased stress in a downward spiral of depression. So, in short – more attention "outward" leads to more meaning and positivity, while more attention "inward" (on the self) tends to lead to less meaning and more negativity.

Dr. Fredrickson has done extensive research on the changes that occur at the subconscious level when people are in a positive frame of mind, and she is convinced that positivity actually works to "rewire" the brain through the process of neuroplasticity in a way that reflects her model of positivity. In other words, positive experiences change our brain's wiring in such a way that makes it more susceptible to *additional* positive experiences. Other researchers have found that being in a positive frame of mind results in improved learning and skill acquisition, and increased access to inner resources such as creativity and mindfulness. People in a positive frame of mind are more easily able to see the "big picture," and find creative solutions to problems by "thinking outside the box." Positivity has also been shown to increase rapport and communication between individuals. Research in the field of psychoneuroimmunology (the study of how the mind, neurology and immune systems affect each other) demonstrates that positivity by itself decreases stress and inflammation, probably by stimulating the parasympathetic nervous system, which causes the heart rate and blood pressure to decrease. Even the blood level of cortisol, a stress hormone, decreases.

One of the most interesting findings in Dr. Fredrickson's work is that happiness or positivity is nonlinear. It has a "tipping point." In her extensive research, she found a "magic ratio" of 3:1, where the upward spiral of flourishing is initiated and maintained with a ratio of three positive experiences for every negative one. This is very encouraging, because it means that positivity and "happiness" can actually be intentionally cultivated. I will explain how later in the chapter.

Anne's Story

I'd like to share the story of a friend whom I will call Anne, who I met in one of the meditation groups I belong to. When I first met her, she was extremely stressed by both her work and her home life. She worked in the field of information technology and was always called upon at all hours to solve people's computer problems. She felt that she couldn't say no and would work until the problems were solved no matter how long it took. Sound familiar? This is a lot like the situations many medical professionals face.

On top of that, she was trying to take care of her aging mother who lived nearby and was starting to show signs of dementia. She was also newly married and trying to start a family. She felt emotionally and physically exhausted and had frequent debilitating headaches. She told me, "I feel like I'm hanging on by my fingernails. I don't know how long I can go on like this." Those statements are typical of someone who is suffering from burnout.

Anne joined our weekly meditation group and began a daily meditation practice. We talked a little about what was going on with her life and I lent her a CD set that I thought might give her some comfort, as it did to me when I was dealing with a similar situation. It was called "When Things Fall Apart" by Pema Chodron, an American Buddhist nun. She found it so helpful she decided to attend a retreat given by Pema at the Omega Institute, a retreat center in upstate New York.

When she came back from the retreat, I noticed a dramatic change in her. She seemed calmer and more relaxed and actually smiled a lot, which she hadn't done much since I'd met her. She told me, "I learned how to forgive my mother for things she did in the past that she can't even remember now, and at the same time I learned not to be so hard on myself. I feel at peace inside myself and I'm able to think more positively about my future."

Even in the year since the retreat, whenever I saw her at meditation meetings, this positive attitude persisted. In addition, she no longer had frequent migraines. When her mother passed away, she told me, "I'm actually OK with it. I don't know how much she took in, but I felt like we made peace with each other. I don't feel like I left anything unfinished." The last time I saw her she was pregnant and was looking forward to being "the mother I always wished I'd had," and sharing in the adventure of raising a child.

I think this story is a good example of the upward spiral of flourishing that Dr. Fredrickson describes. It all begins with mindfulness, which leads to acceptance, which leads to more awareness of the fullness of life, which increases positivity and triggers and maintains the upward spiral as shown below:

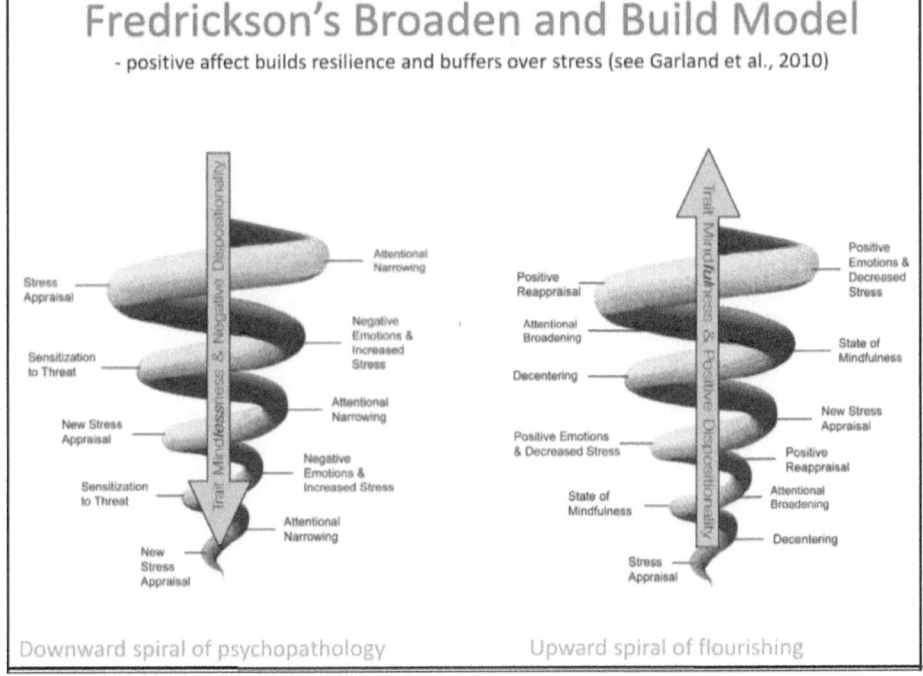

Fredrickson's Broaden and Build Model
- positive affect builds resilience and buffers over stress (see Garland et al., 2010)

Downward spiral of psychopathology   Upward spiral of flourishing

Developing positivity and maintaining the upward spiral

The following is an exercise I do with most of my clients. It is one that never fails to surprise me, in regard to how such a simple exercise can cause such a profound change in outlook and in overall mental and even physical health. This exercise combines the skills of mindfulness and the practice of journaling that you have already read about (and possibly established) and applies them in a specific way to increase positivity and feelings of happiness. Considering the 10 forms of positivity described by Dr. Fredrickson, I have chosen to use gratitude, because in my experience it is one of the more universal feelings. It is also the one that has the most profound effects in a short period of time.

Try this:

1. Think of a time in the last week where you felt genuinely grateful to someone or about something.

2. Describe the event in writing. Who was there? Where were you? What was happening? Describe your experience using all your senses including visual, auditory and kinesthetic (feelings).

3. Why did you feel gratitude? Is there someone who deserves special appreciation?

4. What could you do to have the same or similar experience again?

5. Do the above exercise every day for 2 weeks and see what a difference it makes in your outlook and your mood. You can use it as a substitute for the daily journaling time described in the previous chapter.

Key Points:

1. The search for happiness is a universal human goal, but most people don't know where to look, or fall into the "happiness trap," where the harder they try to be happy, the more unhappy they become. Instead the road to happiness runs through mindfulness and acceptance and finding meaning in everyday life.

2. Happiness is just one aspect of positivity, and there is a "magic ratio" of about 3:1 positive experience to negative experience required to begin and maintain the upward spiral of positivity.

3. You can intentionally cultivate positivity through meditation and journaling.

References:

Amabile T, Kramer S, Harvard Business Review, 2011

https://greatergood.berkeley.edu/topic/happiness/definition

Baumeister R, et.al., J Pos Psych, 2013

Fredrickson, B, *Positivity*, Harmony, 2010

Frankl, VE, *Man's Search for Meaning*, 1946

YOUR *WHY*- VALUES, MISSION, VISION, PURPOSE

Why do you get up every day and go to work as a health care professional? What made you choose a job in the healthcare professions in the first place? Why do you even get out of bed in the morning? Why do you love some jobs and hate others? If you don't have an answer to these questions immediately and clearly, that may be one of the reasons that you're burned out.

In this chapter, we will be exploring your "why" and breaking it down into simple exercises that will bring clarity to your reason for being in the healthcare professions. It will also engender great confidence in your choice to do what you do, where you do it, and with whom you do it. You will find out why you love working in certain jobs and with certain people while you dislike other work environments. This knowledge will empower you to choose the right jobs and work environments and motivate you and those around you to perform at your highest level. This in turn will help to bring satisfaction and even joy into the workplace.

Why your "why" is so important

In the course of doing burnout coaching for physicians, I worked with a research scientist at a leading cancer care hospital in Southern California. I will call him Kevin. Kevin is a M.D./Ph.D., who not only completed medical training and specialty certification in medical oncology, but also earned a Ph.D. in the field of epigenetics, the science of how our environment interacts with our genes to cause certain conditions such as cancer. When we started working together, he was very unhappy in his job. I suggested to him that we explore his values.

I started with the standard values elicitation. I asked him, "What's important to you about career?" Right off the top of his head he said, "Challenge, creativity, independence, honesty, integrity, respect." "What else is important to you about career?" I asked. Next, he said, "financial security, caring for patients, interacting with staff, collaboration." After showing him his list, I asked him to reorder the items in order of most important to least important and this is what it looked like:

Original list:

1. challenge
2. creativity
3. independence
4. honesty
5. integrity
6. respect
7. financial security
8. caring for patients
9. interacting with staff
10. collaboration

Re-ordered list:

1. creativity
2. caring for patients
3. integrity/honesty
4. respect
5. challenge
6. financial security
7. independence
8. collaboration
9. interacting with staff

Then I asked him, "How does your work support or not support your values?" He went on to tell me that he did find the work challenging and creative, but he was under a lot of pressure to do research and publish articles. He felt that the amount of time he had to spend in the laboratory interfered with spending time with patients. In addition, he felt uneasy that some of the money from his grants came from drug companies who stood to benefit from his research. While he conducted his research honestly, he questioned the integrity of his boss in assigning research projects that would most likely benefit the drug companies.

You can see from this coaching conversation how he was able to articulate ways in which his job situation did not support his top three values, which are known as *highly valued criteria*. We then went on to explore ways in which he could arrange for more time in direct patient care. He also talked to his boss about his ethical concerns, and he came away reassured that it was not a problem. At the time that we ended our coaching engagement he was much happier at work, more motivated and energized, and he was setting new goals and action plans that were in alignment with his values. In the next section we will see why working in alignment with your values is so important.

Values drive behavior

Values are our deepest level programming. They determine what you do with your time and how you evaluate the time that you have spent. Other than the most primitive fight or flight reaction, values are the most important driver of your behavior. For this reason, it's important to get to know your values. This can be difficult to do, because values are mostly located in the unconscious mind. The unconscious mind motivates us, determines behavior, and allows us to accomplish the goals we set for ourselves. A problem can arise when the values of our conscious mind, our goal *setter*, conflict with those of our unconscious mind, our goal *getter*.

How do our values drive behavior? Surrounding each value is a set of *beliefs*, which are convictions that we trust as being true. And this core of values and beliefs determine our *attitudes* around any given subject. That attitude is one of the major determinants of our *thoughts and behaviors*.

Where do values come from?

According to sociologist Morris Massey, values are formed during three developmental periods in a child's life.

From age zero to seven—what is known as the *imprinting period*—a child is like a sponge that absorbs everything around him or her and accepts most of it as true. During this period, most of our information comes from our parents or caregivers and our immediate family of origin. The most critical thing that children learn during this time is a sense of right and wrong or good and bad. When there is a disconnect between what we were told as values and what we observe as behavior in our family of origin at this age, it may provide the basis of values conflicts later in life. An example would be a child who is taught that lying is wrong but later witnesses parents or other adults he respects lying to another adult.

The next period is the *modeling period,* which occurs roughly between the ages of eight and 13. This is when we're copying not only our parents but also others around us, including peers at school or in the neighborhood and social or religious leaders. Rather than blind acceptance of their values, we try these values on like a suit of clothes to see how they feel. Children at this age are especially influenced by teachers or religious leaders.

The third period that Massey described is the *socialization period,* which takes place roughly between the ages of 13 and 21. During this time, the largest influence is our peers. As we develop as individuals and question earlier programming either consciously or unconsciously, we turn to people who seem more like us. We're also heavily influenced by media at this age. Nowadays, that means online social media as well as television and print media, and we gravitate to the media which resonates with our values or the values of our peer group.

Although our values are largely programmed by the age of 21, we may add a fourth developmental period that takes place during our 20s and early 30s. During this time, a person is trying on their acquired persona in the context of career, relationship and family, and perhaps modifying their values to some extent.

We have values in each area of life including career, family/life relationships, health and fitness, personal growth and spirituality. Why is it so important for us to know what these are, particularly in the areas of career and relationship?

If we list our values in each area and rank them from most to least important as we will be doing in the following exercise, we typically end up with a list of about 10 values in each area. We refer to the top three values as *highly valued criteria*--and your ability to satisfy those will largely determine whether you're satisfied in each area of life.

For example, if your number one value is not being met or is being trampled in your career, you will probably quit right away. If any of your top three values are not being met, you will be unhappy at your job and will eventually leave. And if two out of three of your top values are being trampled, you will leave sooner rather than later. The same is true for relationship values. If any of your top three values are not being met, you will be unhappy in your relationship and will eventually leave. And if two out of three of your top values are being trampled, you will leave sooner rather than later.

Now that you know how critically important it is to know your values, try the following exercise to help you determine what they are:

Try This:

Use the worksheet in the box following these instructions. First, choose an area of life in which to elicit your values (career, relationships, health and fitness, etc.) You might start with career. Ask yourself or have someone else ask you, "What's important to me about career?" Then make a list of whatever pops into your mind in the first five seconds. Each value should consist of either single word or two or three words-- for example, "integrity" or "having fun". Don't worry about the order; just quickly write down whatever comes to mind in the first five or six seconds. After you have these written down, pause for a few moments before asking yourself, "What *else* is important to me about career?" Then quickly write down the next few things that come to mind in five seconds. And then do a third brain dump: "What else is important to me about career?" And write down the next few things that come to mind. Often, it's easier to do this with someone else asking you the questions and writing down the list.

Once you have all the items written down, look at your list and reorder it in importance, from most to least important. Then rewrite the list in its new order. If some of the words have similar meanings to you, you can combine them into a single value. For example, if "money" and "financial security` mean the same thing, you can combine them. If you're having trouble deciding on the order between two items on the list, *A* and *B,* you could ask yourself the question, "If I could have A but not *B*, would that be okay with me?" And then, "If I could have *B* but not A, would that be okay?"

Once you have finished putting your values in order of most important to least important, make a third column for each value. Here, write down A) "What does it mean to me?" and B) "Why is it important to me?" You can use the worksheet below as a guide.

Now, look at your list of ranked values and look for any conflicts between different values. In other words, would a behavior that supports one value conflict with behavior supporting another value? Finally, check to make sure that each value supports the ones above it on the ranked list.

Area of Life _____

Elicited Values	Reordered Values	What does it mean/ Why is it important?
1	1	1
2	2	2
3	3	3
4	4	4
5	5	5
6	6	6
7	7	7
8	8	8
9	9	9
10	10	10

Now that you have elicited and ranked your values, look at them and ponder the following questions over the next few days. For instance, if the area of life you chose was career, ask yourself, "Does my career as it stands now support my top five values? How does my behavior in career reflect those values?" If you chose relationships, ask yourself, "Does this relationship support my top five relationship values. How does my behavior in this relationship reflect my top five values?"

Your mission, vision and purpose

Anyone who's familiar with business knows that most companies have a mission and vision statement, and some have a purpose statement as well. It's just as important for you to have your own *personal* mission, vision and purpose statements. Being able to articulate your mission, vision and purpose is part of developing emotional intelligence—which is a major determinant of your success in career, relationships or in life in general. Clarifying your own mission, vision and purpose in writing, and posting it where you can see it regularly, can help keep your life in perspective and reduce the likelihood of burnout.

A **mission statement** answers the following questions: What do I do? Who do I serve? How do I serve them? You should write it in the present tense; for example, I might write, "I coach physicians and other healthcare providers using positive psychology and integrative NLP coaching techniques."

A **vision statement** is more generalized and aspirational and reflects where you hope to be in five to 10 years. This should also be written in the present tense, even though it's forward-looking. For example, I might write, "I am a recognized leader in health care coaching, empowering doctors, nurses and health care organizations to manage change, stress and burnout."

And finally, your **statement of purpose**—or what Simon Sinek calls your **why statement**—should be in the following format:

To (the contribution you make to the lives of others) **so that** (the impact of your contribution.)

The statement should be simple and clear, actionable, focused on the effect you'll have on others and expressed in an affirmative language that resonates with you. For example, my purpose or "why" statement might read, "To **transform the lives of healthcare professionals** so that **they can transform the lives of their patients.**"

Take some time and see how this purpose or why statement reflects in your mission, vision, and values. For more information on this process, I refer you to Simon Sinek's book *Find Your Why: A Practical Guide for Discovering Purpose for You and Your Team.*

Now that you know your values, mission and purpose, I encourage you to keep your list of values as well as these statements clearly written out in a place where you'll see them on a regular basis. I keep mine posted directly above my computer monitor in my office. By keeping them prominently displayed, you can regularly ponder the following questions: "Do my behaviors at work (or in relationship, or any other area where I've chosen to concentrate) align with my values, mission, vision and purpose? Do my values, mission, vision and purpose align with the organization in which I work? Do my values, mission, vision and purpose align with those people with whom I'm in relationship?"

Asking yourself these questions will empower you to make powerful and intelligent decisions about what to do in career, in relationships, and other areas of your life.

In the next chapter, we will use the values you elicited, and your mission, vision and purpose statements to make goals that excite and motivate you, and action plans that work.

Key Points:

1. Knowing and clarifying your values using a formal values elicitation process empowers you to make positive and intelligent decisions in career, relationships, and other areas of your life.

2. Your personal mission, vision and purpose statements are highly motivating and can help you prevent burnout.

3. Knowing your values, mission, vision and purpose improves your emotional intelligence, rapport, and communication skills, and increases your likelihood of success in career and relationships.

References:

http://www.ted.com/talks/simon_sinek_how_great_leaders_inspire
_action/transcript?language=en

Sinek, Simon. Find Your Why: A Practical Guide for Discovering
Purpose for You and Your Team. Penguin Publishing Group. Kindle
Edition.

MAKE GOALS THAT WORK

t is now January 5, 2020, and I am finishing the last part of this book's rough draft -- which happens to be chapter 7. When I began writing this book, my goal was to have it finished and to the editor by the end of 2019. Knowing my goal, and the date I did finish, you might think I failed to achieve it-- but I did not. As you read further in this chapter you, will understand why I actually succeeded.

It's no coincidence that this chapter falls in the middle of the book; it's because making and achieving goals is at the center of the coaching process. We will be using all of the knowledge and skills you've gained in the first six chapters of the book as we review the goal setting process. First, you worked on developing the courage to tell your story and to learn from it; then, you learned the benefits of coaching or decided to try self-coaching using the exercises in this book. By developing mindfulness, you'll be able to make thoughtful and considered decisions without being unduly influenced by emotions or limiting beliefs. The habit of journaling will give you perspective, allowing you to articulate your thoughts and feelings and intentionally cultivate positivity.

Perhaps most importantly, the chapter about values led you to discover and articulate your "why," the northern star that guides and motivates you. You elicited and clarified your values in one area of life, and you learned that satisfying your top three values in that area (your *highly valued criteria*) will determine how satisfied you are in that area of life. These discoveries are critically important in the goal setting process, because only when your goals are fully aligned with your values and your purpose will achieving those goals become easier and ultimately more rewarding. You can view aligning your goals, values and purpose the same way as aligning the light in a laser beam: your energy becomes more focused and powerful and directs your actions toward your goal.

After you have set some goals and designed some action plans in this chapter, the second part of the book is designed to give you some more specific skills and tips to help you achieve both your personal and professional goals.

Choosing your goal in one area of life

When choosing a goal, you typically choose one area of your life where you would like to begin. Dividing your life into areas of activity is somewhat arbitrary. Some coaches use 12 areas of life, and some use eight. For simplicity, I divide life into six areas or spheres of influence as shown in the diagram below.

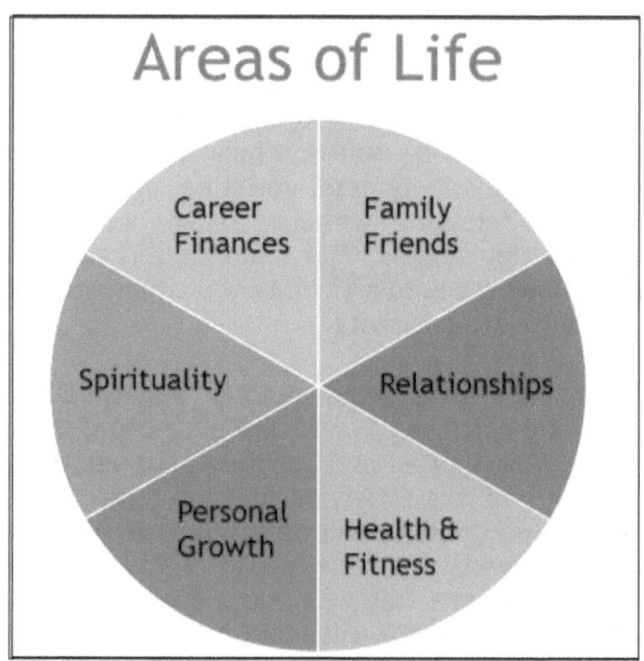

How do you decide with which area of life to begin? One of the easiest ways—and the one which most coaches use—is called the **Wheel of Life** exercise. This exercise has you grade your level of satisfaction in each area on a scale of 0-10 where the higher the number the more satisfied you are with that area of life. You make a mark on the wheel corresponding to the number in each area. Then you connect the dots, which creates a (often lopsided) wheel shape. This visual representation raises your awareness and clarifies which parts of your life are contributing to your well-being and which areas could use improvement. An example from a client of mine who I will refer to as Susan is shown below. After reviewing the exercise, she decided to work in the area of career. I will share her story later in the chapter; but first, let's look at Susan's Wheel of Life below.

As you can see, her satisfaction was lowest in the area of career, with a score 6 out of 10.

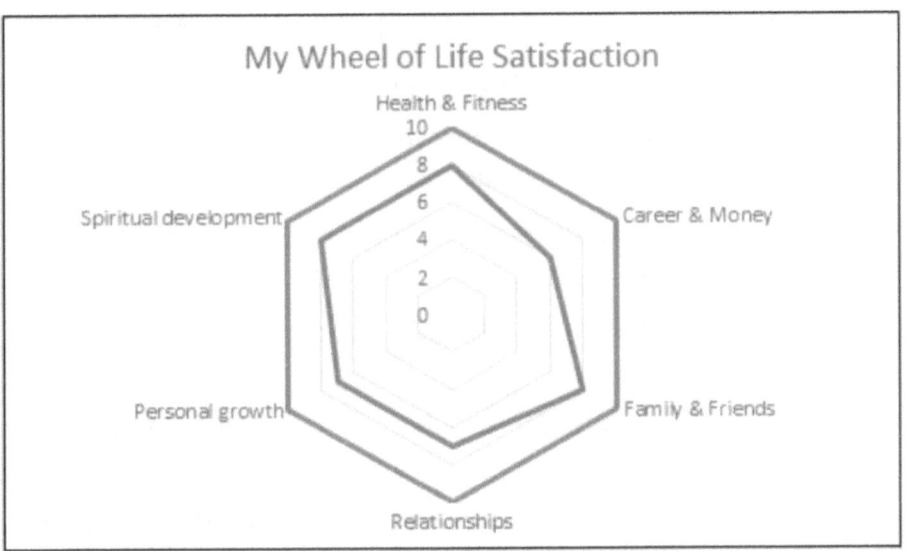

Now it's time for you to make your Wheel of Life using the instructions below and the blank Wheel of Life below the instructions.

Try this:

1. On the blank Wheel of Life make a mark indicating your current level of satisfaction on a scale of 1 to 10 with each area of life.

2. Then draw lines between your marks as shown in the example above.

3. Look at your completed wheel of life and consider some of the following questions:

   a. Does anything surprise you?

   b. How do you currently spend time in each area? How would you *like* to spend time in each area?

   c. Which area would you most like to improve?

   d. Which area, if improved, would make the most difference in other areas of life?

   e. How would you make space in your life for these changes?

   f. What internal strengths and resources could you use?

   g. What external resources or support would you need?

   h. Looking at the above answers, in what area do you want to begin making your first goal and taking action toward that goal?

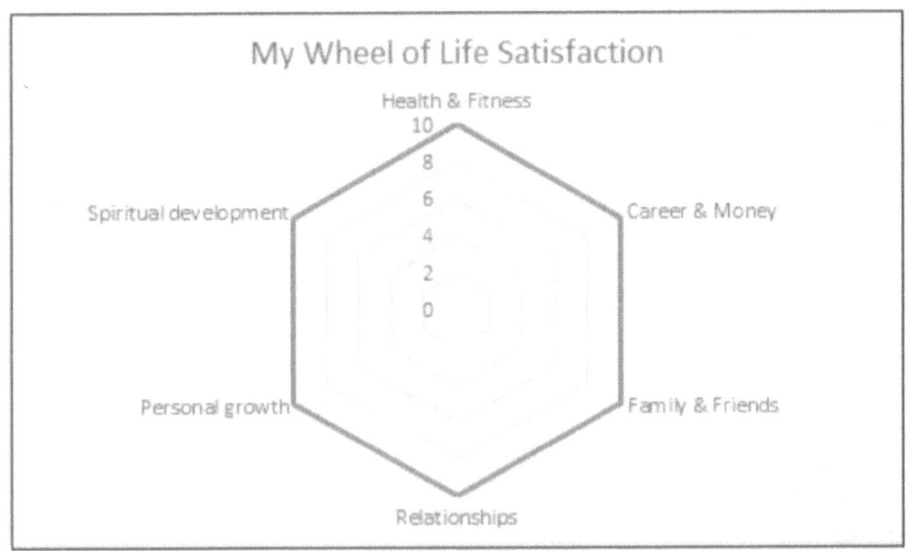

Susan's story

After completing the wheel of life exercise, Susan decided she wanted to concentrate in the area of career. For many years, she had been an aesthetician with her own office doing facials, dermabrasion, massage, acupressure and other holistic aesthetic and healing treatments. She had a devoted group of clients who came back to her office time after time. However, Susan was feeling limited in her practice and wanted to expand. She wanted to offer additional lines of service and products, and she thought the best way to reach out to new clients would be to update her website and social media presence. One of the obstacles that she saw in achieving these goals was that her website and internet infrastructure had always been reliant on the skills of a longtime boyfriend with whom she had an on-again off-again problematic relationship.

As we began to structure her goals and her action plan, discussion of this relationship kept cropping up in our coaching sessions. In fact, for the first two months of our coaching engagement, that relationship is what we spent most of our time working on. This is actually quite typical of some coaching engagements: the client chooses an area of life in which she would like to make progress but feels stuck in that area by problems in other areas of life. It wasn't until we resolved her relationship issues that we were able to make significant and rapid improvements in her career. We discovered together that her values in the area of career including openness, honesty, and integrity were being undermined by her boyfriend's lack of honesty and integrity in the relationship and her continuing to go along with it. Once she was able to align her values (and jettison the boyfriend), she was much happier and began to make rapid progress.

Part of the coaching process with Susan involved helping her to discover and articulate her "why." As it turns out, her purpose as she described it was to "make people feel beautiful inside and outside." At some point during our six-month coaching engagement she decided that one way of doing this was to become a coach herself, since she was already essentially doing coaching work when she talked with her clients. She decided to take a coaching course to learn the specific skills and structures of coaching and now has a successful coaching career in addition to her aesthetic practice.

Motivation and goal setting

An important part of making and achieving goals is not only aligning your values and your purpose with your goals, but also determining what motivates you. Motivation may be positive or negative. An example of a person with positive or "toward" motivation is a student who studies hard in order to excel at a subject. A student with negative or "away from" motivation studies to avoid failing. One way of assessing your motivation is using the values elicitation process we used previously and adding to it.

The following exercise will help you determine whether your motivation is primarily positive or negative. If the area of life that you want to work on first is the same one in which you did the values elicitation, you can use that list of values. If you would like to work on a different area of life, you should elicit your values in that area of life.

Try this:

1. Choose the area of life in which you would like to start making and achieving goals. Use the questions in the Wheel of Life exercise to help you make that decision.

2. Then elicit your values in that area by asking yourself or having someone else ask you, "What's important to me about (that area of life)?" List everything that pops into your mind for the first five seconds. Repeat the process three times or until you have a list of 8 to 12 values.

3. As before, reorder and renumber the list to reflect the order of importance to you from most important to least important.

4. Elicited Values   Reordered values

   1   1

   2   2

   3   3

   4   4

   5   5

   6   6

   7   7

   8   8

   9   9

   10   10

5. Now make a list of what you would consider the opposites of those values.

6. And think about your motivation. Out of 100% of your motivation, what percent is *toward* the value? What percent is *away* from the opposite? For example, if your number one value is wealth and the opposite is poverty, you may be 90% motivated toward wealth and 10% motivated away from poverty; or only 20% motivated toward wealth and 80% motivated away from poverty.

Reordered values	Opposite	%Toward/%Away from
1	1	%/ %
2	2	%/ %
3	3	%/ %
4	4	%/ %
5	5	%/ %
6	6	%/ %
7	7	%/ %
8	8	%/ %
9	9	%/ %
10	10	%/ %

Here are examples from two of my clients:

Client BH was working on health and fitness:

Values	Opposite	% Toward/% Away
1.Longevity	1.Short life	100%/0%
2.Feeling beautiful	2.Feeling ugly/unworthy	90%/10%
3.Feeling confident	3. Lack of confidence	80%/20%

You can see that most of her motivation is **positive.**

Client CB was working on career:

Values	Opposite	% Toward/% Away
1.Greater purpose	1.No purpose	80%/20%
2.Happiness	2.Sadness	40%/60%
3.Stability	3.Instability	10%/90%

You can see that much of CB's motivation is **negative**; that is, avoiding sadness and instability tended to outweigh her desire for finding greater purpose.

Why does that matter? Client BH was successful in her goals of weight loss and has made other positive changes, including getting a better job and buying her first house. Client CB has drifted from one temporary job and housing to another out of fear of instability and sadness. Although she now has a good temp job and rental apartment, she still doesn't feel a sense of purpose in it. In short, positive motivation tends to spur on more lasting changes, and extend to other areas of one's life whereas negative motivation tends to get us stuck. Let's explore the relationship of motivation to goal attainment in the diagrams below:

When your motivation is primarily negative (to move away from something undesirable) *as shown in the figure below,* you are trying to get away from an undesired state or pain. But when you get far enough away that the pain or discomfort decreases, you lose motivation and drift back toward the undesired state until the discomfort increases enough to motivate you to move away again. So, you tend to bounce up and down in the grey zone where things are OK but not great or terrible, which means that you tend *not* to reach your goals.

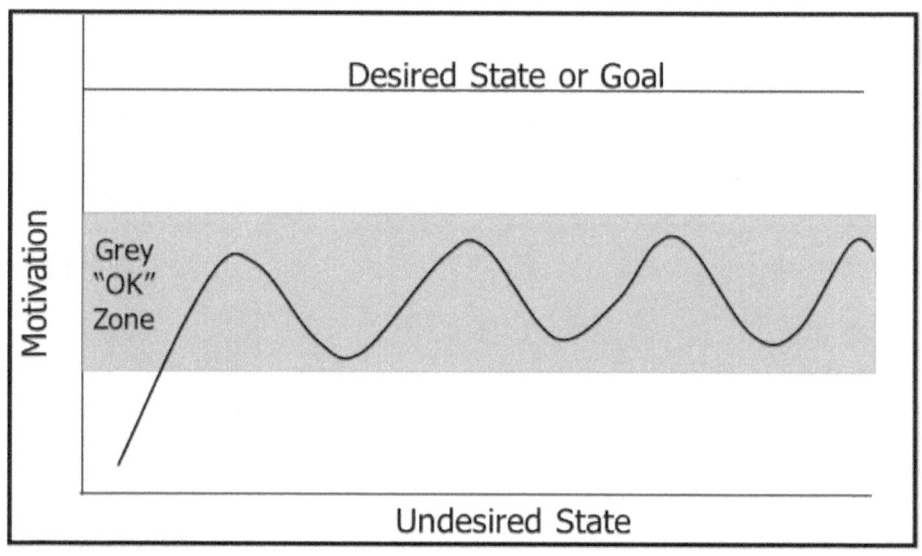

When your motivation is positive (toward your goal), your motivation stays high and only starts to diminish as you approach your goal *as shown below.* The way to keep motivation high is to set intermediate goals. Then when you reach 90% of the first goal and motivation starts to taper off, you set a new, higher positive goal and motivation again increases as shown in the figure below. I tell my clients to, "Celebrate at 90% and set a new goal." Both the celebration and the new goal produce positive motivation. That's why I celebrated getting 90% of my book finished and set a new goal of getting it formatted and published by the end of January.

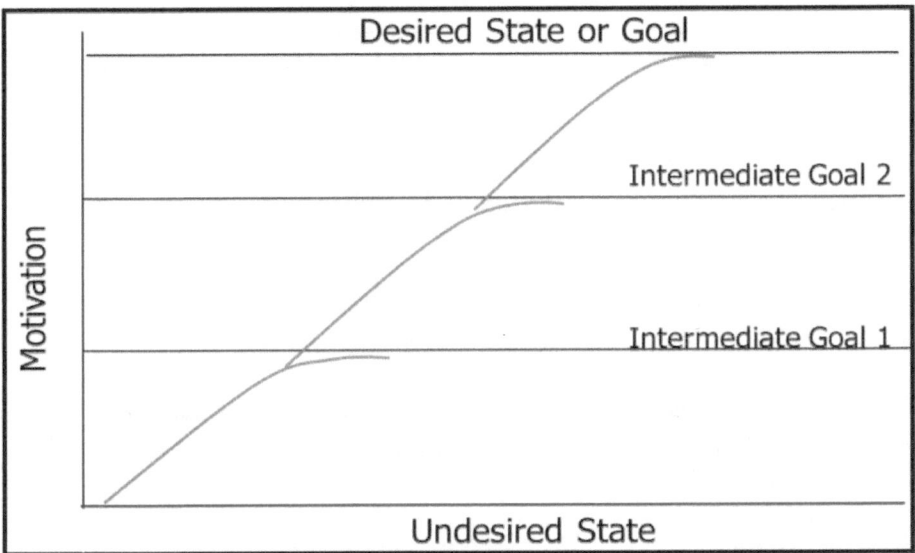

S.M.A.R.T. Goals

In addition to making sure that your goals are aligned with your values and your purpose, and that your motivation toward the goal is positive, it is important to set goals that are challenging enough that they will stretch your abilities—but not *so* difficult that they are overwhelming or impossible. The way that we do that is through the use of S.M.A.R.T. goals. S.M.A.R.T. is an acronym that describes how to put your goal into writing in a way that makes it achievable and leads to an action plan. That's important, since it is said that "a goal without a plan is just a wish."

S.M.A.R.T. goals are always written in the present tense and have a specific timeline. An example would be, "It is now January 31, 2020, and my book is published on Amazon." Let's see how that goal fits into the S.M.A.R.T. goal acronym:

S: The goal as written is *simple* and *specific*.

M: The goal is *measurable*. This particular goal is binary; that is, either I completed it, or I didn't. Other goals may be measurable in units such as dollars, number of times something is done, distance etc.

A: The goal is written *as if now*, and also *achievable* because I know of people in a similar situation who have accomplished similar goals. And finally, it is a goal that could *affect all areas* of life.

R: The goal is *realistic* and *results focused*. It is also *responsible*. That is, it is good for self, good for others, and good for the community.

T: The goal moves me *toward* my aim and my purpose. It is *time-bound* with a specific completion date that adds a sense of urgency without being overwhelming.

Now it's time for you to write your own S.M.A.R.T. goals using the following questionnaire. Decide on an area of life, and keep in mind your purpose and your values in that area of life. Write a S.M.A.R.T. goal for one year from now, three months from now, and one month from now.

S.M.A.R.T. Goal Questionnaire

Goal: It is now (time/date) _____

And   I am(doing/being/having)_____

Simple. Specific. What will the goal accomplish? How and why will you accomplish it? What will it do for you or allow you to do?

Measurable. Meaningful. How will you measure whether or not the goal has been reached (list at least two indicators)?

As if now. Achievable. Affect all areas of life. Is it possible? Have others done it successfully? Do you have the necessary knowledge, skills, abilities, and resources to accomplish the goal? Will meeting the goal challenge you without defeating you?

Results-focused. Realistic. Responsible. What is the reason, purpose, or benefit of accomplishing the goal? What is the result (not activities leading up to the result) of the goal? Is it good for self, others and the community?

Time-bound. Toward your Aim. What is the established completion date and does that completion date create a practical sense of urgency? Does it align with your purpose and your values?

Make an action plan

As I said above, "a goal without a plan is just a wish." After writing your goal, you then need to formulate a plan to achieve it. An action plan can be written in one of two ways: either forward or backward. If you have a fairly good idea about how to get to your goal, it makes sense to write it forward. Ask yourself the question, "What is the very first thing I have to do to move toward my goal?" Then ask yourself, "After that, what is the very *next* thing I have to do to move toward my goal?" And then continue on until you reach the goal.

Current State_____

	A	B	C	D	E
1	What has to happen?	What do I need to do?	What resources do I have or need?	Priority	Target date for objective
2					
3					
4					
5					
6					
7					
8					
9					
10					
11					
12					
13					
14					x

SMART Goal_____

If the action steps and timeline are not as clear to you, it may be helpful to move backwards from your goal. Ask yourself, "What is the very last thing that has to happen, or I have to do before I reach my goal?" Then ask yourself, "in order for that to happen, what has to happen or what do I have to do just before that?" Then proceed backwards stepwise to the present moment. Choose one of your goals and try making an action plan using the action plan form above.

The power of habits

Sometimes the biggest thing preventing you from taking the necessary steps to achieve your goal is the intimidation of getting started. What can you do when procrastination or a lack of motivation is standing in your way? You can turn to the power of habits. An action that is a habit doesn't require any particular motivation. All it requires is a trigger to set the automatic behavior in motion. Author James Clear has written a book entitled *Atomic Habits* on how to make new desirable habits and how to break old unproductive ones. Below is a summary of Clear's four laws to create a good habit (this information is also available on his website at https://jamesclear.com/atomic-habits/resources).

The first law: Make it obvious. First, become aware of your current habits—both good and bad ones. If you want to install a new habit, it may be helpful to link it with another good habit that you already do. This is called habit stacking, where the old habit acts as a trigger for the new habit. Another way to start a new habit is simply to write down your intention and post it somewhere prominent. I have posted on my mirror, "After breakfast, meditate" and "Before bed, journal." The action I want to do (meditate) is paired with something I know I'm not going to forget to do (breakfast.) And the notes are posted where I'm sure to see them when I brush my teeth in the morning and evening.

The second law: Make it attractive. You can pair a behavior that you want to do with one that you already do, especially if it's enjoyable. Or you can put yourself in an environment that supports that behavior. For example, you are more likely to exercise if you go to the gym or even buy a new pair of sneakers.

The third law: Make it easy. Design your environment to make the new action easy to perform with the minimum number of steps. Automate as much as possible to reduce the effort involved. For example, I have a specific desk and laptop in my study that is always set up for writing articles or books. I invested in a high-quality microphone and transcription software so that I only use the keyboard to make corrections. Writing is much easier for me when I dictate instead of typing, so I am more likely to sit down at any time and dictate a paragraph or two.

The fourth law: Make it satisfying. Reward yourself immediately when you complete your habit. Keep track of your habits in a way that you can see easily so that you can try to keep a habit streak going. If you forget to do a habit, make sure that you never miss twice. That way, you get back on track immediately.

Remember: break down all of your action steps to small manageable pieces. Make sure that you congratulate yourself or give yourself a virtual high five every time you complete a step before you move onto the next one. Breaking a large task into smaller micro-tasks makes it seem less daunting. My favorite example is climbing Mount Whitney, the highest peak in the lower 48 states—something that I've done a number of times. It is a very long and demanding day hike, covering 22 miles round-trip and reaching an elevation gain of 6000 feet. There is one particularly steep section that ascends over a series of 99 switchbacks. If I stand at the bottom of that section and look up at the tiny people at the top, I find it overwhelming. So I don't count the switchbacks; but every time I reach the end of one, I give myself a pat on the back before starting the next one. It makes the climb less psychologically challenging. As the saying goes: "A great journey begins with a single step." I would add, "The journey continues with another single step, and another, until you reach your goal."

In chapters 1-6 you did the necessary self-exploration to make goals that work and that motivate you. In this chapter you learned how to make S.M.A.R.T. goals and action plans. In the next chapters you will learn some more advanced tools that can transform those goals and plans into reality.

Key points:

1. Making and achieving challenging goals is central to the coaching process.

2. Setting goals that work requires that you align your goals with your purpose and your values in any area of life.

3. Positive motivation (moving towards something you want) is more successful than negative motivation (moving away from something you want to avoid) in reaching your goals.

4. All important goals should be written as S.M.A.R.T. goals. You can use the worksheet in this chapter if you forget what the acronym stands for.

5. Make an action plan for your goals. A goal without a plan is just a wish.

6. If procrastination or lack of motivation stop you from making progress toward a goal, use the power of habits to move forward.

Chapter 8

RAISE YOUR EQ

D o you know what *your* EQ is? First: do you even know what EQ stands for and why it's so important? You'll learn how developing your EQ—or emotional intelligence, as it's often known—helps you understand yourself, your behaviors, and helps you manage your behaviors in the most productive way. Emotional intelligence also helps you understand and empathize with others and manage others in a team approach. In fact, EQ is even more important than IQ in determining your career success. So, how can you measure your EQ, and how can you improve it? I'll answer all these questions and more throughout this chapter.

The term **"emotional intelligence"** was first described in a 1964 paper by psychologist Michael Beldoch. The first published use of the term "emotional quotient (EQ)" and comparing it to IQ was in the British journal *Mensa* in 1987. However, the term emotional intelligence achieved wide popularity after the publication of a 1995 book by psychologist Dr. Daniel Goleman entitled *Emotional Intelligence-Why It Can Matter More Than IQ.* This bestselling book was followed up by many additional articles and books on the topic. EQ or emotional intelligence is thought to be an ability—one that, unlike IQ, we can study and improve over time. IQ is considered to be a trait which does not change over time, and therefore cannot be improved significantly.

There's currently no completely accepted model for a testing emotional intelligence, but there are some widely accepted assessments, including the Mayer-Salovey-Caruso Emotional Intelligence Test (MSCIT) and the Bar-On EQ-i. The Emotional Intelligence Appraisal® is another popular test of emotional intelligence authored by psychologists Drs. Travis Bradberry and Jean Greaves.

Why is emotional intelligence so important?

Emotional intelligence, or EQ, is a fundamental or foundational set of competencies and, according to Dr. Bradberry, is "so critical to success that it accounts for 58% of performance in all types of jobs. It is the single biggest predictor of performance in the workplace and the strongest driver of leadership and personal excellence." No longer is job performance based solely on productivity or economic factors, but as Dr. Daniel Goleman puts it, "We are being judged by a new yardstick, not just how smart we are or by our training or expertise, but also how well we handle ourselves and each other."

Emotional intelligence, which is related to rapport and effective communication, is critically important in the field of medicine. Studies have correlated the degree of physician empathy and rapport directly with patients' clinical outcomes. Even in studies of objective measurements such as diabetes control, patients of physicians who score high on empathy and rapport had significantly better control of their diabetes as measured by differences in hemoglobin A1C. So, whether you're a doctor or a nurse, your EQ and ability to improve it are critical not only for your own well-being at work, but also for your patients' well-being. In fact, three of the seven critical competencies required by the Accreditation Council for Graduate Medical Education (ACGME) for medical students are "interpersonal and communication skills," "professionalism," and "interprofessional collaboration"—all of which are connected to your emotional intelligence.

EQ is not IQ.

IQ, or cognitive intelligence, appears to be unrelated to EQ. IQ appears to be fixed at birth, or at least as early as testing can be instituted. It is not flexible and can't be changed by training. IQ measures your ability to learn. Although there have been some ethical arguments about whether there is cultural bias in the standardized tests that are currently used to measure IQ, we do know that your IQ predicts relatively well how well you will do in school and your ability to score on standardized tests of academic achievement. However, IQ is a relatively poor predictor of success in one's job or life.

In contrast, emotional intelligence is "your ability to recognize and understand emotions in yourself and others and your ability to use this awareness to manage your behavior and relationship." Emotional intelligence, as measured by various tests, is also not the same as personality type, which is also more fixed for an individual and is usually measured by the Minnesota Multiphasic Personality Inventory (MMPI). Personality, like IQ, is considered a trait, not an ability. Although you might expect people with the personality type including the trait extroversion to be associated with a higher EQ, this is not the case. EQ tends to be independent both of IQ and personality type.

People with high EQ are more successful. According to Dr. Bradberry, based on results of testing with the Emotional Intelligence Appraisal®--at least in the business world--"people with the highest levels of intelligence (IQ) outperform those with average IQ just 20% of the time, while people with average IQs outperform those with high IQs 70% of the time." Let's look at the four skills that are considered parts of emotional intelligence: **self-awareness** and **self-management**, which make up **personal competence**, and **social awareness** and **relationship management**, which make up **social competence.** The way these elements fit together is outlined in the diagram below.

Social and Emotional Competencies		
	What I Observe	*What I Do*
Personal Competence	**Self Awareness**	**Self Management**
Social Competence	**Social Awareness**	**Relationship Management**

Personal competence

Self-awareness refers to your ability to perceive and understand your own emotions in the present moment as they relate to specific events or people. Interestingly, Dr. Bradberry found that only 30% of the people he tested were accurately able to identify their emotions as they happened. Self-awareness is a critical skill; without it, you are the victim of your emotions instead of the master of them. Self-awareness is so important to your success that 83% of people who test high in self-awareness are top performers in their field, and just 2% of the bottom performers test high in self-awareness. Interestingly, Dr. Bradberry found that the people in business with the highest self-awareness scores were direct managers of people, as well as human resources professionals. High-level corporate officers, including CEOs, often had lower EQs and lower self-awareness scores.

The second part of personal competence is self-management, which is based on self-awareness. This is your ability to be aware of your emotions and to stay *flexible* enough to be able to direct your behavior positively. The brain's frontal lobe executive function prevents what is commonly known as "amygdala hijack." This occurs when the flight-fight-or-freeze instinctive behavior triggered in the amygdala, the most primitive part of the brain, results in irrational or overreactive behavior.

Social competence

The foundation of social competence is social awareness: your ability to identify emotions in other people and understand what is going on with them at the emotional level. It requires that you separate what you're feeling from perceiving what the other person is feeling. This skill depends on having enough personal awareness and self-management to listen to and perceive another person's verbal and nonverbal communication, without feeling the need to insert your own emotions into the conversation. Nurses tend to have a relatively high social awareness; sadly, physicians are often lacking in this skill.

And finally, there is the second part of social competence: relationship management. It is built on all three of the above competencies and is your ability to use both your awareness of your own and others' emotions to manage your own feelings and to successfully navigate your interactions with others. Relationship management builds rapport and emotional bonds between people. This bond is a result of the quality of the interaction and the depth and time you spend interacting with the other person. Lack of relationship management often results in conflict at work or at home and is a major cause of personal stress.

What emotional intelligence looks like to other people

Although emotional intelligence assessments can provide a score that you can use to work on your skills, sometimes the best indicator of EQ is what other people say about you. Here are some examples from Dr. Bradberry's most recent book:

"What **Self-Awareness** Looks Like:

Dave T., regional service manager. High self-awareness score = 95*

What people who work with him say: "Dave has clear long-term goals, and he doesn't make sacrifices for short-term gains. [He] is an 'upfront' kind of guy who doesn't play 'mind games' with people. I have witnessed this at company meetings and in meetings with customers. In short, Dave manages his emotions; they don't manage him. I've seen him accept difficult business news with a brief frown, and then he quickly moves beyond that and partners with his team to find solutions to improve the situation."

Tina J., marketing manager. Low self-awareness score = 69

What people who work with her say: "On occasion, Tina [pushes her] stress and sense of urgency onto other people. It would be good for her to better understand how her behavior affects others' work and emotional stress. Also, she sometimes comes across as defensive or aggressive, so for her to be more aware of her tone and language would be helpful."

What **Self-Management** Looks Like:

Lane L., healthcare administrator. High self-management score = 93

What people who work with her say: "Lane is the epitome of patience and understanding during heated, emotionally-charged meetings. Others around her become fully embroiled in the discussions, and Lane actively listens and responds with knowledge and wisdom." "I have seen first-hand how well she deals with difficult situations (i.e., termination of an employee). Lane is sensitive, yet direct and to the point. She listens patiently and sets a high standard of conduct."

Jason L., information technology consultant. Low self-management score = 59

What people who work with him say: "In stressful situations, or when something goes wrong, Jason sometimes responds too quickly, sharply, or disjointedly. I wish Jason would take some time to cool off and slow down before responding. He's so emotional. I have seen his coworkers respond in disbelief to the manner in which he communicated with them. Jason means well but can panic when he is stressed. His reactions trickle onto his teammates."

What **Social Awareness** Looks Like:

Alfonso J., pharmaceutical sales manager. High social awareness score = 96

What people who work with him say: "Alfonso has a rare talent to be able to read [others'] emotions very well. He adjusts to different situations and manages to build relationships with almost anyone. Good examples are dinners, meetings, and ride-alongs with reps."

Craig C., attorney. Low social awareness score = 55

What people who work with him say: "Craig needs to allow others to feel good about their ideas, even when he has a better plan. He also needs to be more patient and allow them to have equally effective plans that are just different from his plan. I would like him to seek to understand what people are feeling and thinking, and notice what evidence there is regarding situations before speaking his opinion or offering solutions."

What **Relationship Management** Looks Like:

Allister B., physician. High relationship management score = 93

What people who work with him say: "Allister is a wonderfully patient, empathetic listener, which is why his patients love him. He tries very hard to be nonjudgmental and gives people the benefit of the doubt. He is the same way with the nurses and technicians. I've seen Allister in situations where his patients' families were asking difficult questions, and he was able to remain calm and answer without alienating the family member asking the questions. He listens carefully to what others say and never shows if he is upset or bothered by it. He responds kindly but with authority."

Dave M., sales manager. Low relationship management score = 66

What people who work with him say: "Dave always reacts to people rather than responding to them. To have a strong opinion is fine, but to dismiss others' thoughts is not. He also needs to tailor his communication style to the person. His approach is nearly always very direct, which can be difficult for some people to handle."

Building your emotional intelligence

As I stated at the beginning of the chapter, we can all improve our emotional intelligence (EQ) with practice. The personal competencies I've described are most easily developed by practicing the first two skills covered in this book: mindfulness and journaling. It can be helpful to remember that an emotion is simply energy in motion and is therefore constantly changing. It arises, peaks, and then fades away. Emotions are a combination of two things: a thought, or thoughts, and a sensation somewhere in the body.

The more we practice mindfulness, the more aware we become of our thoughts and our sensations, and how they arise, peak, and fade away naturally. We learn as part of the process of mindfulness not to hold onto nor reject any of these thoughts or sensations, but simply to observe them in a neutral fashion. In much the same way, the self-management component of personal competency comes when we allow the thought and sensation to diminish or go away before we take any action. This allows our actions or words to therefore more likely be a result of thoughtful consideration. We consider the likely effects of those words or actions on others, which encompasses the skills of social awareness and relationship management.

Awareness of other people's feelings and successful management of relationships is often more difficult under stress. You must therefore become acutely aware of when you're under a significant amount of stress and use a mindfulness technique during these moments— such as the single-breath meditation, or even temporarily removing yourself from the stressful situation before you overreact. Some people use the simple technique of counting to 10 while taking some deep breaths, or even just deciding to put off reacting until after getting a night of sleep. It may be helpful to talk to a non-involved person to get another perspective on the situation. You want the purpose of that conversation to be to learn about yourself and what the other person may be feeling—not to air your grievances, which tends to reinforce the problem. I will discuss more about the social competence skills in the chapter on rapport and communication.

Know your strengths- Eliminate Imposter Syndrome

Do *you* ever feel like other people in your profession know a lot more than you do, or are much more highly skilled? Do you have a persistent internal self-doubt or fear of being exposed as a "fraud?" Additionally, do you ever feel sometimes that you do not deserve the success you have achieved and attribute it incorrectly to simple luck or to faking it? Thoughts like these signal the presence of **"imposter syndrome."** While people across professions can feel this way, doctors and nurses—despite lots of external evidence of their knowledge and competence—experience this phenomenon frequently.

The term imposter phenomenon, or imposter syndrome, was first described in 1978 in high-achieving women. However, subsequent research has shown that the prevalence of imposter syndrome is essentially equal in men and women. This phenomenon often coexists with feelings of generalized anxiety, depression, and low self-confidence, which is why imposter syndrome is closely associated with burnout. The imposter syndrome is a product of our personality, our upbringing, and our educational system, particularly in medical education. As we've talked about before when discussing the causes of burnout, some of the deeply held beliefs that we acquire during medical training are partially to blame. These include the fear of failure, the Superman/Superwoman complex (where you think you have to be able to do anything by yourself), and the unspoken rule to "never show weakness."

The figure below shows schematically, the misperception that causes us to feel less competent or knowledgeable than other people. We tend to magnify other people's strengths and underestimate our own as shown on the left. The reality is shown on the right. Everyone has their own unique set of strengths, which may or may not overlap with yours. So, the comparison of your strengths with someone else's is simply not relevant. What is important is to use your strengths in just the right amount and to improve areas where you may not be as strong. Coaching can help with this.

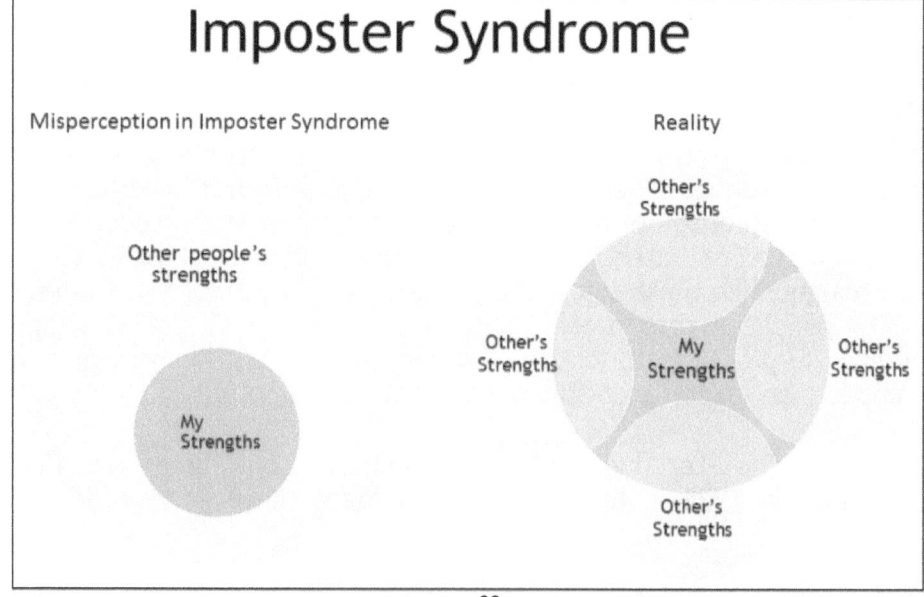

Imposter Syndrome

Misperception in Imposter Syndrome

Reality

Other people's strengths

My Strengths

Other's Strengths

Other's Strengths

My Strengths

Other's Strengths

Other's Strengths

Imposter syndrome can be attacked at two different levels. One is at the unconscious level using techniques such as hypnosis, neurolinguistic programming, or mental and emotional release (MER)®. Individual or group therapy may also be useful but tends to take longer and works primarily at the conscious level.

I use NLP techniques in breakthrough sessions with individual clients. However, with most clients and with groups, I tend to use **strengths assessments** as a shortcut to eliminate the imposter syndrome at the conscious level. First, I have the client take the VIA Survey of Character Strengths (which you can take free at https://www.viacharacter.org/,) which is one of the two most commonly used strengths assessments, and the one I prefer. This assessment measures 24 different character strengths which have been found to be universal across countries, cultures, and belief systems. These character strengths are core positive capacities for thinking, feeling, and behaving in ways that benefit oneself and others. I then have clients look at their top five strengths, which are known as the **signature strengths**, and recognize where in their lives they have used or could use these strengths in ways that benefits themselves and others. This helps them realize that their capabilities do very much exist, and that they have been calling on them for years.

One of the biggest problems with imposter syndrome is that people tend to underestimate their own knowledge, skills, and strengths, while tending to overestimate those of others. If you look at your own VIA personal strengths, or even your top five signature strengths, simple mathematics will show that your chance of having the same exact signature strengths in the same order as another person is approximately 1 in 10 billion. In other words, your particular set of strengths is essentially unique—making comparison with anyone else irrelevant. Your goal should be to utilize *your* signature strengths to the right degree, and to develop other strengths that are further down your list. I find this approach much more useful than simply trying to reframe the experience psychologically or to make a list of the client's personal accomplishments.

Key Points:

1. Emotional intelligence (EQ) is more important than IQ in determining your success in life.

2. Whereas IQ is a trait which is fixed early in life, emotional intelligence or EQ is an ability which can be measured and improved intentionally.

3. Many intelligent and high achieving individuals suffer from "imposter syndrome." One of the best ways of dealing with it is knowing and utilizing your individual signature strengths, which are unique to you, and recognizing that comparison with others is meaningless.

References:

Bradberry, Travis. Emotional Intelligence 2.0 . TalentSmart. Kindle Edition.

Goleman, D. (1998). Working with emotional intelligence. New York: Bantam Books

Mayer, J., Caruso, D., & Salovey, P. (2000). Selecting a measure of emotional intelligence: the case for ability scales. In R. Baron-On & J.D.A. Parker (eds.): The handbook of emotional intelligence (pp. 320-342). New York: Jossey-Bass.

Hojat M, et.al., Academic Medicine, Vol. 86, No. 3, March 2011, p359

https://globalleadershipfoundation.com/geit/eitest.html

https://www.viacharacter.org/character-strengths

Chapter 9

LEARN TO COMMUNICATE EFFECTIVELY

Odds are, you think you already know how to communicate. After all, you talk to people every day. You text message. You post on Facebook and Instagram, and if you're old like me, you even send emails. What I'm going to cover in this chapter is *effective* communication—that is, communication that elicits a specific desired response from the other person and that results in improved rapport and empathy between two people.

Why are empathy, rapport, and communication so important for healthcare professionals? Good communication skills reduce conflict and friction in the work environment – and professional conflict has been shown in both physicians and nurses to be a major risk factor for burnout. Effective communication results in better patient care and satisfaction, and it is also necessary to promote teamwork and increased efficiency in the workplace as we will see in the chapter on teamwork.

Communication can change the world

In chapter three, I introduced you to my spiritual teacher, Zen master Thich Nhat Hanh. It was his work trying to bring peace to Vietnam in the 1960s that prompted Martin Luther King to nominate Hanh for the Nobel Peace Prize. While he didn't win the Nobel that year, he *was* awarded the very first Gandhi-Mandela Peace award in recognition for all he has done to bring peace to the world in 2019.

In 2001, Hanh began an initiative to establish a peaceful dialogue between Israelis and Palestinians in the Middle East. Groups of about 30 Palestinians and Israelis were invited to Plum Village Monastery in France for two weeks of meditation, mindfulness practice and conversation. In order to promote effective communication, the participants first meditated together and then practiced the type of active listening that I will be discussing in this chapter. You can see from the participants' comments what a difference this experience made in their lives.

As one Palestinian said, "Something happened quietly and with deep listening that helped me to be in touch with each person's pain and suffering. I would like to see us continuing what we have done here in Israel and expand it. I learned two important things here... to listen deeply, without rejecting the other person and his or her point of view, even if it was difficult for me to hear, and I learned how to share especially difficult feelings and experiences in a calm and respectful way, so that the other person would listen. *We were not trying to find solutions but rather understanding and support.*"

According to an Israeli, "Being exposed to terror, violence, and denial every day, whether you are Palestinian or an Israeli, makes it hard to stay in touch with your tenderness and softness, makes it hard to open your heart and not put on a suit of armor, and makes it hard to be able to forgive and to ask for forgiveness. Each one of us, in our own lives, and all of us together, are trying to help each other to do that. *During the Dharma discussions, we try to create an atmosphere of openness and support, in which we can learn to speak with love, without blaming and to listen deeply.* Even though we all suffer, we can slowly start to feel the rays of gratitude, gently warming us."

It is truly amazing what the practice of mindfulness, active listening, and compassion did in this scenario. It resulted in communication that allowed people who were mortal enemies to begin to understand each other. Just imagine what the world would be like if we could all cultivate our mindfulness and compassion and learn how to communicate as effectively as these two groups did. The good news is – we can. And you can start with yourself.

Rapport is essential to effective communication

You've probably heard the word "rapport" before—but do you know what it is, and why it's so important? Before you can begin to communicate effectively with another person, you have to develop rapport with them. Rapport is an attitude of mutual understanding and empathy that makes communication possible or easy. Studies have shown that a clinician's ability to develop rapport with a patient or client may be a **more important** factor than the practitioner's actual medical knowledge or clinical competence in patient outcomes. One of the reasons for this is that the physician's empathic communication skills influence **patient satisfaction** and **patient compliance**. And as we all know, patient compliance is critical in achieving good clinical outcomes. One study from the Journal of Academic Medicine compared the empathy scores of physicians with their diabetic patients' blood sugar control as measured by their levels of hemoglobin A1c. This study actually showed that patients of physicians with higher empathy scores had significantly better control of their diabetes.

In order to understand how to rapidly develop rapport, you need to know that only 7% of our communication is the **words** we speak. 38% is in **how** we speak—that is, our loudness, tone, timbre (quality of voice,) and inflection. The other 55% of our communication is **nonverbal,** reflected in our physiology, including our posture, gestures, facial expressions, proximity to the other person, and even such things as how fast we breathe and how rapidly we blink. To develop rapport, you also *need to understand how the other person experiences their world.*

Sensory perception and your model of the world

As discussed in the chapter on coaching, neurolinguistic programming (or NLP) is the science of how our experiences are expressed in our language. The NLP communication model is based on the assumption that everyone experiences the world through their five senses. The experience, or the memory of the experience, is stored in the brain in areas specific to those senses.

It is estimated that we experience up to 5 million bits of sensory information per second, but the **conscious mind** is only capable of processing about 126 bits of information per second. So, what happens to the rest of the sensory information? Fortunately, the **unconscious mind**—that part of the mind which works without our conscious awareness—is capable of processing approximately 2 million bits of information per second. The excess 3 million bits or so is filtered out before it even gets to the brain, based on our state in the moment and on what our previous experiences have deemed important. The figure below summarizes this process.

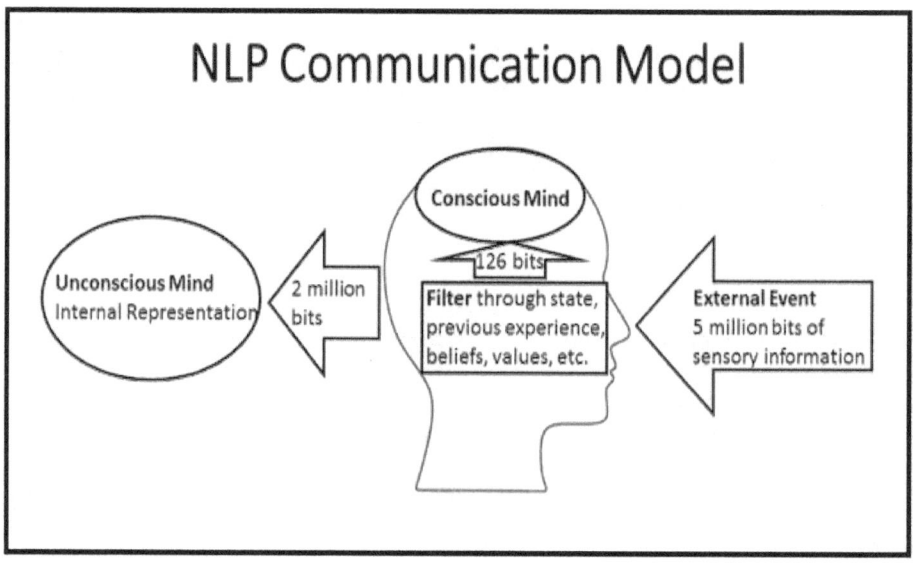

You can see how this process would have been useful to the earliest *Homo sapiens* when they lived on the savannas of central Africa. An early man who had previously encountered a lion might be temporarily alarmed by tan-colored rock in the rough shape of a lion while scanning his surroundings. His mind would unconsciously register a possible threat and begin the "fight or flight" reaction before his conscious mind could analyze the image as a "rock." His earlier experience of a lion, including the sight, sounds, smells and feelings of the moment, were stored in his unconscious mind in what is referred to in NLP as **an internal representation.** The unconscious nature of this reaction was critical to survival. If he had to think about it consciously his reaction would have been much slower, and he might have been eaten!

The NLP model also explains why different people have different experiences of the same events. For example, my brother and sister have completely dissimilar memories (internal representations) of events that took place in our childhood. It's almost as if we didn't even grow up in the same family. Chances are, you've had a conversation with someone where you've both recalled the same event in your own unique ways – maybe a recollection of a fight with a significant other, or a memory of a meeting with a colleague. Knowing that different people have different experiences and memories of a given event is a very powerful concept. In NLP terms, it means that everyone has their own particular **internal model of the world.** *Respecting another person's model of the world and trying to understand it is the foundation of building rapport.*

Primary representational systems

NLP also recognizes that while we have five senses, human beings experience the world primarily through their visual (sight,) auditory (hearing,) and kinesthetic (feelings) senses, and one of these senses may be dominant for a given person. The dominant sense for any individual is called their **primary representational system**, and it is reflected in the language they use. A person who is predominantly **visual** may use words such as, "it looks like...," "appears to me...," "I can envision...," or "it's clear..." An **auditory** dominant person might say something such as, "it sounds to me like...," "it's music to my ears," "that rings a bell," or "I hear you." The **kinesthetic** dominant person might say something such as, "it feels right to me...," or "I need to get a hold of that," or "that touches me," or "that seems solid." These words are called **linguistic predicates.**

Developing rapport rapidly

It's important to understand these concepts because **people tend to like people who are like them.** You can rapidly develop rapport with another person using the processes of **matching** and **mirroring**. First, you listen carefully to your patient or client – both to what they say, and how they say it. Are they predominantly visual, auditory or kinesthetic? Try matching their primary representational system by using choosing words that fit with that modality. For example, you could begin a sentence with a visual person by saying, "It looks to me like..." An auditory person might respond well to, "It sounds to me like..." To a kinesthetic person, you could say, "That feels like..." You can also try matching some of your client or patient's tonality, timbre, rate of speech and some of the key words they use. Observe his or her posture, their physical mannerisms, their proximity to you, whether they are leaning in or back, and some of their gestures. Matching means copying some of their postures, mannerisms and movements. Mirroring is like matching, but as if they were looking in a mirror. For example, when they cross their left leg, you would cross your right leg.

Of course, you must be subtle when you do this, or the other person will notice consciously and think that you are mimicking or making fun of them. One very subtle matching/mirroring technique that I learned from studying the great psychiatrist and hypnotherapist Dr. Milton Erickson is matching my breathing rate to my client's, or even tapping my finger in time to their blinking. This process of matching their verbal and nonverbal communication is picked up by their **unconscious mind,** and results in rapid rapport.

How can you tell if you're in rapport?

One indicator of rapport is that your patient or client may say something like, "I feel comfortable with you," or "I feel like I can really talk to you," or even, "I feel like we've known each other for a long time." If you're really paying attention, the most reliable indicator of rapport is a **change in physiology**, either in the client's or in yours. If you closely observe your patient while you're talking to them, you may notice that they become more relaxed when you're in rapport. Their facial tone decreases, and their skin looks shinier. Their color may shift from light to slightly darker, and they may lean toward you more. If you're aware of your own feelings, you might notice a sense of warmth or possibly some tingling. One of the best indicators of rapport is that the other person starts to match some of *your* postures, words, and tonality.

Hearing is not the same as listening

Sir William Osler, known in the medical world as the godfather of the clinical examination, had this to say: "Observe, record, tabulate, communicate. Use your five senses. Learn to see, learn to hear, learn to feel, learn to smell, and know that by practice alone you can become expert." Or as one of my professors used to say, "If you listen carefully to the patient's history, they will tell you the diagnosis." Even in this day of advanced medical diagnostics and electronic health records, listening to the patient or client is still one of the greatest skills that a healthcare practitioner can have.

90% of what I do as a coach is active listening, and most of the remaining 10% is asking a few select powerful questions. This section will summarize several ways of listening and asking questions that come from the arenas of coaching, therapy and NLP.

The most important element of what we call **active listening** involves being present 100% and paying attention to the client or patient. Your **mindfulness practice** will really help you with that, and there are a few other elements to keep in mind. You should ideally be sitting at the same level as the other person and facing them at about a 90-degree angle, or directly facing but offset about a chair's width to the right or left. You should **not** be multitasking or doing anything other than listening and perhaps taking some brief notes on what the other person is saying. And even if you are taking notes, you should be making eye contact with the patient. Don't stare; but try to take in their whole face and body in your visual field. That will allow you to more easily pick up any changes in their physiology which indicate being in or losing rapport.

The second element of active listening is to defer judgment, even in your thoughts. You should be listening, not thinking about what you're going to say next. The third aspect is to listen to the **context**, not only the content, of what's being said. In other words, to "listen between the lines." Does their tone of voice and body posture agree with the meaning of their words? For example, a person may say, "I agree with you," while they lean back in their chair and cross their arms across their chest which is a non-verbal signal that they *disagree* or are putting psychological distance between you.

In order to stay in rapport, the patient or client needs to know that you are listening to them and that you understand them. There are different ways of responding that allow the speaker to know that you've really heard and understood them. These techniques are based on "client-centered" therapy developed by Dr. Carl Rogers, one of the best-known psychologists of the mid-20th century.

The first possible response is **simple reflection**. In reflection, you repeat or paraphrase back to the client **in their own words** what you heard them say. For example, the client may say, "I'm really worried that these symptoms mean that I have cancer." A reflective statement from you might be, "What I'm hearing from you is that the symptoms really worry you." Then the client or patient may elaborate further or may correct you if you didn't understand what they meant.

Summarizing is another form of reflective listening, where you take several statements that the client has made and summarize them back. For example, if the patient says, "I know that my blood sugar and my blood pressure are too high, and my father died of a heart attack when he was 60, so I'm really worried I might be developing heart disease. And these chest pains worry me." Your summary reflection might be, "You have some risk factors and a family history of heart disease, so you're worried about these chest pains."

Other types of appropriate responses involve asking questions for clarification, getting more details about something they said, or opening new topics of discussion. Most of these questions should be **open-ended**, which means they begin with the words **"how"** or **"what."** Some examples are, "I hear that you're worried that your heart disease is going to affect your employment. How exactly is it going to interfere with your work? What do you think could to happen with your job?" Or you could simply say, "Tell me more about that." Sometimes a simple nod and "mmm-hmm" is enough to let them know you're listening.

Regardless of how you respond, you should follow the **80-20 rule**: the client or patient should be doing the talking at least 80% of the time and you should only talk 20% or less. Also, **don't be afraid of silence**. You have to give the person time to mentally process before they talk, since many people have not had this kind of conversation before. It's also critical to keep in mind that kinesthetic people talk and process more slowly. It's as if they have to "feel out" the words. My rule is to allow at least 5 seconds of silence (or longer if it's comfortable) before I say anything else.

One of the most challenging situations you can face as an active listener occurs when the client or patient says something and expects you agree or disagree with them. Fortunately, you can use the **agreement frame here** to maintain rapport. The agreement frame is a two-part sentence linked by the word **"and."** This is how I use it: When I actually agree with the client's statement, my response is, "I **agree** with you, **and** ..." If the client or patient says something with which I don't agree fully or disagree, I say "I **appreciate** that, **and** ..." If they make a statement with which I disagree, I will say, "I **accept** that you believe that, **and** ..." I use this sentence construct to perhaps bring in another point of view without outright disagreement, which would break rapport. The most important thing is not to use the word **"but"** in your sentence. When you use the word "but" in a sentence, it negates the first part, so that if you say, "I agree with you, but....," it essentially means, "I don't agree with you."

Use the following exercise to practice your listening skills. Practice using open ended questions and remember to follow the 80-20 rule. While you're conversing look for linguistic predicates to determine whether they are predominantly visual (seeing,) auditory (hearing) or kinesthetic (feeling) in the words they use to describe their experiences. Then try using words that match their preferred sensory modality. Look for opportunities to try out the agreement frame.

Try this:

1. Get together with a friend or family member and ask them to name a person that was a role model or influenced their life in a positive way.

2. Ask them questions about that person and how that person influenced them using open-ended questions starting with **"what"** or **"how"** for about 10 minutes.

3. Practice active listening and try some **reflective** responses.

4. Subtly pace your subject (without telling them what you're doing) by **matching** some of their posture, positions, tone, speed of talking and the **preferred sensory modality** of their linguistic predicates.

5. Look for **signs of rapport** like change in skin color from light to dark, relaxed facial muscles around eyes and increased shininess of the face, pupils slightly constricted, and decreased breathing rate.

Motivational Interviewing

Motivational interviewing is a variation of client-centered counseling, developed by psychologists Drs. William Miller and Steven Rollnick to help clients change negative or self-destructive behaviors and adopt more positive ones. This technique is particularly useful for physicians, nurses, and health and wellness coaches, because we know that 80% of chronic illnesses that we see are related to unhealthy lifestyles and nutrition. However, it's often challenging to get people to break those habits and adopt healthier ones.

The approach you take will be determined by how **ready** the client or patient is to make the needed changes. According to the research of two psychologists, Drs. DiClemente and Prochaska, there are **five stages** that adults go through in order to change behavior. In the first stage, **pre-contemplation**, they are either totally unaware or in denial of their problem behavior. Most patients you see will be in the second stage, **contemplation**; this is where they know that their behavior is causing health problems, but they're not yet ready to change it. This stage may last from 6 months to a year or more. The next stage, **preparation,** is where the patient starts exploring the different options to change their behavior. This stage is shorter, often 3 months or less. The next stage is **action**, where the patient actually changes their behavior in a positive way. And the last stage is **maintenance,** which is maintaining the behavior consistently.

Motivational interviewing works particularly well in the contemplation phase; in this stage, the patient understands that their behavior is unhealthy and is going to cause them problems in the long run, but they're not sure if they really want (or are able) to change. This internal conflict results in a feeling of **ambivalence.** Motivational interviewing takes advantage of that feeling of ambivalence to move them toward action. The skills that you use are the ones you already learned—including active and reflective listening, affirmation, and summarizing—in a way that **amplifies the ambivalence** and moves them toward readiness for change.   The key points are in the pneumonic OARS: Use **O**pen-ended questions. **A**ffirm whatever positive statements they make and healthy behaviors they already have. **R**eflect back their concerns about the effects of their unhealthy behaviors. **S**ummarize their statements to make them more obvious.

Here is an example of what a motivational interview might sound like from the **practitioner's** side:

"How has your diet of soda and potato chips affected your health?" (open-ended question)

"What are your concerns if you keep eating like this?" (open-ended question)

"I hear you say that you're worried about getting diabetes and heart disease and not seeing your kids or grandkids grow up. What could you do to change that?" (summarize, open-ended question)

"You say you've started walking 3 miles every day. That's great! How is that improving your well-being?" (reflective listening; affirmation; positive open-ended question)

A critical component is to find out how prepared they are to change and encourage them to **move to the next level of readiness:**

"When do you think you will be ready to change your diet in a way that supports your health? Three months? Great! Here is some information about diet and exercise to help you get started. Let's make an appointment in two months to work out a plan."

And here is **my all-time favorite** motivational interviewing question:

"On a scale of 1-10, how likely are you to make these changes? You said 7. Why not 5 or 4?"

This might seem strange -- but suggesting a number on the scale **below** what they say forces them to justify why they need to make the changes and moves them toward readiness. You can follow this up with, "What would it take to move you from a 7 to a 10?"

Non-violent Communication improves relationships

In his book *Nonviolent Communication*, author and psychologist Dr. Marshall Rosenberg says, "While studying the factors that affect our ability to stay compassionate, I was struck by the crucial role of language and our use of words. I've since identified a **specific**

approach to communicating in both speaking and listening that leads us to give from the heart, connecting us with ourselves and with each other in a way that allows our natural compassion to flourish. I call this approach nonviolent communication, using the term nonviolence as Gandhi used it. While we may not consider the way we talk to be violent, words often lead to hurt and pain, whether for others or ourselves."

You may want to read his book in its entirety; but I'm going to present an outline of how to use nonviolent communication, **NVC**, to improve your relationships at work and at home. This is important because the quality of those relationships is one of the factors that can either drive or reduce burnout.

There are four components to NVC:

1. **Observation-** When somebody does or says something that affects us in an emotional way, we need to be able to observe our feelings and to articulate to the other person exactly what behavior or statement that they made that triggered these feelings in us.

2. **Feelings-** We need to take responsibility for our own feelings, observing them clearly and stating in a nonjudgmental or evaluative way exactly what we're feeling.

3. **Need-** We state what needs of ours are connected to the feelings that we have identified and are honest in expressing those needs.

4. **Request-** We ask the other person in a polite way to change their behavior or speech in a very specific way that will meet our needs.

The first part of NVC is to make observations in ourselves and to be able to communicate them verbally or by some other means to the other person in a **nonjudgmental** way. The second part of NVC is to **receive** the same four pieces of information from others while remaining mindful and compassionate. We are sensing what they are observing, feeling, and needing **without reacting** ourselves. Finally, we are hearing their request and deciding whether or not we can fulfill it.

To simplify, the template for an interaction using nonviolent communication could sound like this:

When you **say/said** or **do/did** _____, I **feel/felt** _____ because I **think/thought** _____.

I **need** _____, so please **say/do** _____.

Here's an example of using NLV:

"When you don't respond to what I'm saying, I feel sad because I think that you don't value my input. I need to feel valued in a relationship, so please respond when I'm talking to you."

You can see in the above example of NVC how the person is making a simple observation of their experience, while at the same time taking responsibility for their own feelings and the thoughts that triggered those feelings. The second part is expressing the need that is not being fulfilled and requesting specifically how the other person could satisfy that need.

Compare this with the way most people communicate:

"You always ignore what I say" (generalization; assumes that the other person heard and understood) "You make me so mad!" (does not take responsibility for own feelings and the underlying thought process or assumption.) Or, "I wish you would take me seriously." (does not clearly state a need and the specific action desired). Comments like these are vague and not very helpful, and don't get to the heart of what has bothered this individual – and what they'd prefer instead.

I urge you to try using this type of conversational process both at work and at home. You may initially get a negative reaction, especially if you have previously been judgmental or blaming in your communications. However, if you persist you will find that others around you start to adopt the same type of speech—leading to improved rapport and communication.

Now that you've learned the importance of rapport and communication with your patients, coworkers, bosses, spouses, children, and anyone that you come into contact with, the next chapters will describe how to utilize those skills to develop your team, and reduce friction at work and at home so that you can work less and enjoy life more.

Key Points:

1. Having rapport with your patients or clients improves their satisfaction as well as their outcomes.

2. Rapidly developing rapport is a skill which you can practice and develop.

3. Active and reflective listening are the keys to effective communication and to getting the most important clinical information from your patients.

4. Motivational interviewing can help patients give up unhealthy behaviors.

5. Using the Non-Violent Communication model can improve your relationships at work and at home.

Reference:

Rosenberg, Marshall B. Nonviolent Communication: A Language of Life, 3rd Edition: Life-Changing Tools for Healthy Relationships (Nonviolent Communication Guides) Puddledancer Press. Kindle Edition

Chapter 10

TECHNOLOGY, TEAMWORK AND TIME MANAGEMENT

I put these three items in the chapter title's together not just because I love alliterations, but because how well you use the available technology and your health care team are key factors in how effectively you manage your time. When energy flow in your team and information flow in your EHR (electronic health records) goes smoothly, the whole day seems more effortless and everyone gets to go home on time. Large-scale studies from Mayo Clinic showed that the incidence of physician burnout increased from 45% to 55% between 2011 and 2014—a time period that coincided with widespread adoption of EHR. The latest study in 2017 found that the average physician spent about half their workday and an additional 28 hours per month on nights and weekends completing EHR tasks. At the same time, both patient facetime and physician satisfaction decreased.

Electronic Health Records: Be a Lover, Not a Hater.

Do you spend 50% or more of your time inputting or reviewing data from an EHR system? Does data input and correction cause you to go home late most nights? Do you find yourself finishing up your documentation from the day in the evening after dinner? In this chapter, I will be showing you how you can use the technology, instead of the technology using you.

One pundit claimed that many doctors spend 50% of their time working on the EHR system, and 50% of their time swearing at it. I know that some systems can be very frustrating to use and there is a great temptation to swear. However, swearing is not a good utilization strategy. So instead, I'll show you how to develop a strategy that works for you, so that you can do adequate documentation and still get home on time and have your evenings to spend with your family.

The strategies that I'm going to discuss here are general ones, rather than approaches for dealing with a specific system or manufacturer, since there are so many players in the field. If you are on the outpatient side, you will most likely be dealing with Epic, Allscripts, GE or Athenahealth as top vendors. On the inpatient side, you may be dealing with Cerner, Epic, McKesson, Meditech, and a host of other providers. Of these, Cerner (Siemens) slightly dominates the inpatient market at the moment, while Epic has equal dominance in the inpatient and outpatient market. But why does this matter?

I'll explain from the point of view of a diagnostic radiologist. In radiology, we had the fortune (or misfortune, depending on your perspective) of leading the healthcare profession into the digital age. Many radiology practices including mine went digital 25 years ago, as the number of images from a single study such as a CT scan ballooned from 24 images per patient to hundreds of images per patient encounter. This is when it became obvious that we could no longer look at images on physical pieces of film. Fortunately, at that point, the output of many imaging machines went from analog to digital, and that digital data could be stored on a central server and viewed quickly and efficiently at computer workstations.

It took a few years for demographic data such as patient history, diagnosis and other clinical information to be stored on a RIS (radiology information system) and for that data to be seamlessly married to the image data on the PACS (picture archiving and communication system). Those four or five years of being half digital and half analog were very frustrating, as standards were worked out between the major providers. Eventually, the systems became more seamless and user-friendly, and radiologists were able to do more work in less time than before. The two factors that made the biggest difference to our efficiency was learning how to utilize the systems to their highest potential by becoming power users, and by giving feedback to the vendors in a constructive way so that they could improve their products.

For the last five years, many clinicians have found themselves in the same situation that we did early on in our adoption of digital imaging. That is, systems are designed by engineers and billing departments, with clinical utility added on as an afterthought. However, I now think we're at the end of the transition period and at a point where many systems are actually in a position to help us manage our patients *and* improve patient care. So instead of feeling used by the system, you can use these systems to your own advantage.

The best way to become a power user of an EHR system is first to take whatever training is available to you from the vendors. If it doesn't sink in the first time, take it a second time. The second major tip is to look around you at other clinicians and see who appears to be least frustrated and spends the least amount of time doing the documentation. Then spend some time with them to see how they do it. Look at their workflow and what shortcuts or work-arounds they found useful.

The following are some tips that may be helpful on your system.

1. Focus on the home screen and optimize it so the you have the most useful information available to you with the fewest mouse clicks. Set the filters to present the most important clinical information to you when you first open a patient record.

2. Use templates and macros for repetitive types of procedures or diagnoses. It's usually much better to copy a template from a power user than to try to make your own up from scratch.

3. Make a personal favorites folder for common medication, admitting or other orders, so that you can easily retrieve and reuse them. Put the folder on your home page.

4. See if your system has the ability to translate the data you enter into a correct diagnosis code. If it doesn't, look for some third-party software that can do so.

The most challenging and time-consuming part of documentation is the progress note that requires free hand input. The most important thing to remember is that you're not writing the great American novel here. You should not duplicate any information that is included elsewhere in the record; however, **I strongly recommend against cutting and pasting because it tends to propagate previous errors.** Instead, briefly describe any changes that have taken place since the last encounter. Specify your treatment plan and your rationale for that plan in the fewest possible words. You don't even need to use complete sentences as long as you're providing clear information. Of course, all of the above only applies if you are the unfortunate one that has to do all of the data entry. Ideally, most data should be pre-populated or entered by someone else such as a scribe or medical assistant. This is where you need your team—and I'll talk more about teamwork in the next section.

People often ask me what to do about all the pop-up messages that you receive on the screen from doctors, nurses, pharmacies and even patients. Trying to answer every message as it comes up distracts you and splits your attention. Despite what many believe, your brain is *not* capable of multitasking. When you think you're multitasking, your attention is actually shifting back and forth between different tasks—and you end up paying less attention to *everything*. The best strategy in most cases is so set aside all messages and answer them in a batch twice a day. At that time, you can determine which messages are most important and answer those first. Many messages do not require a response. Lab and x-ray results can also be dealt with in twice-a-day batches. Routine prescription refills should be handled by a nurse if possible. Again, teamwork and communication are key. If you just can't ignore the pop-ups, cover that part of the screen with a Post-it-Note.

Put down the smartphone

How often do you check your smartphone during the day—and how much of that time is directly related to performing your professional duties? Do you know how many total minutes per day you spend on your smartphone? While these devices' have increased our ability to communicate with each other and have the potential to improve our lives and the lives of our patients, there are negative effects of too much smartphone usage on individuals and their social and family relationships. There is no doubt that smartphones and the apps that run on them are designed to capture and hold our attention; even app designers admit this. There is a new code in the DSM-5 manual which identifies addiction to internet gaming as a disorder, although addiction specifically to smartphones or social media are not yet categorized as disorders. There is, however, a correlation between the amount of smartphone and social media use among adolescents with comorbidities of anxiety and depression.

So, while it is convenient to be able to access urgent messages from your coworkers and even your family, studies have shown that there is often a gap between what different providers consider urgent. Additionally, too much smartphone usage negatively impacts interprofessional relationships as well as patients' perceptions of physicians' professional behavior. In addition, the use of smartphones to retrieve confidential patient information in various locations may not meet HIPAA standards for confidentiality. This fact coupled with an increased prevalence of patients secretly videotaping their physicians leads me to believe, and advise, that **smartphone use be banned in the examination room and in the consult room.**

How do you balance the positive and negative effects of smartphone use during the other times in your workday? I would suggest treating the smartphone as just another computer at work. Except for emergency phone calls, all communication should be batched about twice a day, including returning or forwarding important text messages and emails and deciding whether to answer voicemails. You should undertake these communications in a private location. It's just as important to set some rules for this kind of communication when you are *not* at work. When dealing with work-related calls or texts after hours, it is very important to clearly specify your boundaries, and let people know that you will respond to non-emergency communication the next business day, and that people should not expect immediate replies.

Of course, is up to each individual to decide how much they want to engage on social media at home. However, the use of social media at work should be strongly discouraged. For one thing, it distracts from patient care and may result in more errors. Studies have also shown that overuse of social media apps and smartphones in general can be deleterious to your social and family relationships. If you're concerned that you might be overusing your device, both Apple and Android-based phones now have built-in trackers to determine how much screen time you spend every day, including a breakdown of what apps you are using. These devices allow you to limit your own screen time. It's ironic, to say the least, that apps like Facebook and Instagram now offer ways to track and limit your usage voluntarily while their algorithms continue to provide an experience designed to attract compulsive use.

Finally, there is evidence that use of smartphone and other LED screens that emit blue light wavelengths can interrupt the onset of normal sleep and even alter sleep patterns. As we'll see in the next chapter, getting a good night's sleep is the foundation of your physical and mental health. For that reason, many experts recommend that you limit screen exposure in the two hours before bedtime.

Who's on your team?

All medical care is delivered by teams. Your team is comprised of the people you work with every day. Depending on the setting, it may consist of doctors, nurses, allied healthcare professionals such as PA's, nurse practitioners, pharmacists, other clinicians, and the support staff. In an outpatient office, your team includes everyone responsible for the care of your patient from the time they walk into the door until the time they leave, including schedulers, front office, back office, and technical staff. For example, as a radiologist with a multi-office outpatient practice, I was in two or three different locations during the week. In each location, my team consisted of one other radiologist, a nurse, multiple imaging technologists, the schedulers, front office staff, medical records and patient transporters.

It's critical to know who is on your team. Identifying and working with team results in improved communication, better productivity, increased safety, and a better patient experience. Your main tool for improving teamwork is the **team huddle meeting**. Although this practice began in the corporate world, it has direct applications in healthcare.

General rules for a team huddle are:

1. Start on time, end on time and keep it short (five to ten minutes). Keeping this meeting timeboxed and productive is essential to its effectiveness.

2. Include the right people. If the entire team is too large, a representative from each part of the team should attend.

3. Have a simple agenda that requires you only share *essential* information. There should be no complex problem solving, detailed explanations, or airing of grievances. A typical team huddle agenda includes celebrating yesterday's successes, establishing today's priorities, and addressing potential obstacles.

Your first decision is who will attend the team huddle. In a clinic or large office, there should be one representative from each area. For example, on my team, I had the nurse, one scheduler, the front office manager, the medical records manager, the chief technologist in MRI and CT, the main technologist in women's imaging and the technologist doing special procedures and fluoroscopy.

Then, identify who is going to run the huddle. In my situation, the doctors rotated offices; but because the same nurse was present in one office for the week, she was therefore designated team leader. Have the huddle meeting in a convenient, neutral area, not in your office. Our team meetings were held in the nurse's station. Decide as a team what time to hold the meeting. You may choose to hold one huddle first thing in the morning, or a morning and afternoon huddle (which makes sense in an outpatient office,) or at change of shift, as we did. The specific time of the huddle should be designated, and the team members need to understand that (except for medical emergencies) attendance on time is expected. Everybody stands; after all, this is supposed to be a short meeting.

Begin the meeting by noting something that went well the day before or recognizing a person who did something beyond their duties for a patient or another staff member that day. The way we did this was to have a small box in the main hallway with a pad of small sticky notes next to it. Anybody who wants to commend somebody for special kindness or patient service during the day makes a quick note of the person's name and what they did and puts it in the box. Somebody may be commended for a helping a patient or for helping out a co-worker without being asked. Before the team huddle meeting, the team leader selects one or two of these notes randomly to present at the beginning of the meeting. (It is important to spread the love around even if not everyone gets the same number of positive notes.) It may be corny, but I gave the day's special person a sticker to wear that says, "You're a Star!" or "Team Player," or "Thank You!" I also ordered small packets of custom M&Ms with the same words to give out.

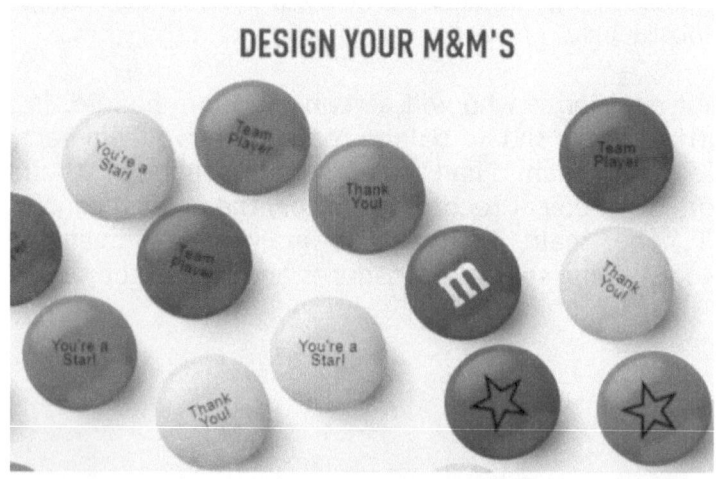

Next, we looked at the schedule and identified any particular challenges that were likely to arise and identify who was (voluntarily) going to take care of the problem. This is also a good time for any team member to ask for help with anything coming up during the day. Finally, we reminded ourselves and recommitted ourselves to our purpose for being there. It may be the purpose as stated in the company mission and vision statement; or the team can make their own purpose statement to commit to for that day. Committing to a common purpose results in better team alignment and productivity and assures that everyone starts their day on a positive note.

Two case studies in the use of technology and teamwork

First, I'd like to tell you how technology and teamwork improved the efficiency and the quality of care in my own practice. It began with the ordering process. Physicians or their representatives could enter imaging orders directly online through our physician portal. We integrated the computer assisted ordering decision support tool from the American College of Radiology into our platform. Using this tool assured that the patient was getting the right study at the right time for their particular clinical presentation. It also captured much of the patient demographics for our information system. Our scheduling department used this information to contact the patient and schedule the examination. When the patient arrived at the office, the front desk staff collected additional demographic information, which was entered directly into our system using either computers or iPads. The patient facilitator took the patient to the changing area, then to the nurse's station if an IV was to be started, and finally to the appropriate imaging modality area. The imaging technologist double checked the clinical information and elicited additional clinical information from the patient and entered that information into the patient record.

When the imaging procedure was finished, the patient facilitator accompanied the patient back to the front desk and helped get him or her check out. While this was happening, the technologist attached the imaging study to the demographic data in the RIS-PACS system on the central server. Then the appropriate subspecialty radiologist for that imaging study could retrieve all of the demographic information, clinical information, and images from any one of our seven offices. The transcription of the dictated report was done by word recognition software with a final editing by a human transcriptionist. The radiologist could review and sign reports electronically, almost immediately for emergencies and in batches for routine studies. The reports and images were then available online to the ordering physicians on the physician portal. This type of efficiency increased radiologist and technologist productivity, and patient wait times were decreased.

Another excellent example of using teamwork and technology to share the load and to decrease burnout was developed by Dr. Corey Lyon at the University of Colorado Family Medicine Clinic. In his own words, this office used "advanced team-based strategies such as team-based documentation, pre-visit planning and testing, and an expanded scope of practice for medical assistants and nurses." They also utilized "team-based and motivational interviewing and coaching, and delegation of certain elements of chronic disease care, preventative care, medication reconciliation and refills, and acute care to staff using standardized protocols. These strategies were designed not only to reduce provider burnout, but also reduce staff burnout by ensuring that they could grow professionally and engage more intimately in patient care."

Lyon called this program APEX (standing for either Ambulatory Process Excellence or Awesome Patient Experience.) A critical element of this process was expanding the role of the medical assistant. This individual went from simply rooming the patient and taking vital signs to a more complete role, including staying with the provider in the exam room to provide additional documentation and findings as a scribe, preparing orders to be signed, and preparing patient instructions. The MA also became responsible for entering lab orders, scheduling follow-up, and escorting the patient from the office at the end of the visit. While making the medical assistant essentially a patient concierge might seem like an extravagance, Lyon's team found was that due to the system's increased efficiency, the cost of the additional medical assistants required was actually offset by the savings that came from increased patient throughput. The providers also made extensive use of EHR templates and standardized clinical protocols. These protocols were developed in a series of eight rapid improvement events (using Lean Sigma procedures) involving over 100 providers and staff members to get buy-in from the whole clinical team.

Other outcomes of this program included improved clinical quality measurements and a better reported patient experience on the exit (CG-CAHPS) survey. This government mandated survey may be used by patients and referrers to select providers and may even impact provider payments. The number of providers and staff reporting burnout and overall dissatisfaction dropped by about 50%. In addition, quality metrics and preventative care improved significantly. Dr. Corey cited as one of the keys to his program's success a **full-time embedded practice coach** who was unaffiliated with management, or any factions within the practice. As a result, this individual was able to resolve any conflicts between staff, supervisors, providers, and leadership.

Now that you know the advantages of working together as a team, and you have the communication skills to facilitate individual and group communication, it's time to assemble your team and get their buy-in by explaining that it will make the work day go more smoothly and get everyone home on time.

Explain the purpose of the team and the rules of the huddle. Remember if you are the doctor or charge nurse or other supervisor, you are an equal member of the team and should not dominate the conversation. Whoever is selected as the team captain should be someone who can keep people on track, firmly but politely.

Try this:

1.Identify the members of your team and get their agreement to work together in huddle meetings. Explain the huddle meeting's structure and purpose to secure their buy-in.

2.Get agreement about when and where to hold your huddles and the importance of beginning and ending on time.

3.Decide who is going to run the huddle (Hint: Not the doctor.)

4.If possible, agree on a statement of purpose (see the chapter on knowing your why for some guidance on this.)

5.In the meeting:

    a. Have the schedule for the day in hand

    b. Check in with everyone and see how they are doing

    c. You may all want to do a single breath meditation to get on the same wavelength (see Chapter 2.)

    d. Celebrate a win from yesterday. If you're recognizing a "star" from yesterday, make sure they are there to receive the   compliment.

    e. Ask the team if anyone sees any potential problems in the schedule, such as a difficult patient or a scheduling conflict.

    f. Team members can suggest a solution or volunteer to help out with a problem. Any team member can ask for help with a specific task for the day.

6.Finish by repeating the team or organization purpose statement and another single breath meditation or other boundary ritual to cement your intention for the day.

Key Points;

1. EHR is not going away. Become a power user by learning about the capabilities of your system from the vendors and other power users in your unit.

2. Take care of non-emergency communications such as messages from patients and other providers in no more than two batches per day. Remember, everyone including you has their own idea of what is an emergency. Clearly communicate and enforce your boundaries firmly but politely.

3. Try to spread out data entry among everyone on the team including admitting, front desk, nursing, and other providers.

4. If you are a physician try to get a scribe or "super MA" to do contemporaneous documentation while you interact with the patient. When dealing with administration, justify the added expense in terms of increased patient satisfaction, improved quality and throughput.

5. Utilize team huddle meetings daily to get everyone on the same page and make the workflow smoother so everyone can go home on time.

References:

Lyon C, English A, Smith P, A Team-Based Care Model That Improves Job Satisfaction;

https://www.aafp.org/fpm/2018/0300/p6.pdf

https://edhub.ama-assn.org/steps-forward/module/2702161 (Imaging clinical decision support)

https://edhub.ama-assn.org/steps-forward/module/2702506 (daily team huddle)

Chapter 11

BALANCE YOUR LIFE: SLEEP, EAT, MOVE, LOVE

As I discussed in Chapter I, I view burnout as an energy problem or energy imbalance. Every day, we make withdrawals from our spiritual, mental, emotional, and physical energy bank account by dealing with life and death issues at work, fighting with our electronic health record software, navigating relationship problems at work or at home, and overcoming lack of adequate sleep or nutrition. We also make deposits into our energy bank account every day, by engaging in activities like meditation, journaling, positive interactions with our peers and our family, and by taking the time for self-care, including eating well, sleeping, and exercising. This chapter will cover this very important element of caring for ourselves so that we can be in the best shape possible for our colleagues, patients and loved ones.

The mind-body energy connection

People used to talk about our minds and bodies as these were two separate entities living inside of us that somehow had to communicate with one another. We now know through studies in psychoneuroimmunology and epigenetics that the mind and body are not only connected; they are completely integrated as a single unit. We know that our neurologic system not only includes the brain, spinal cord, and peripheral nerves, but also the autonomic nervous system, which controls all of our visceral functions, including heart rate, breathing, metabolism, and the entire endocrine system. Even our immune system is in constant two-way communication with the central nervous system. This communication in the mind-body is mediated by energy flow, whether in the form of electrical, chemical, or physical energy.

There is also two-way communication and energy connection between us and the world around us—including other people. In order to maintain a positive balance in our energy bank account, we must constantly monitor our energy state to make sure that we are not always putting out more energy than we're taking in. As we saw in the first chapter, if we consistently withdraw more energy than we deposit, our energy bank account not only goes to zero; it becomes overdrawn, and we run the risk of going into energy bankruptcy or burnout. The figure below illustrates this concept and shows the four interconnected spheres of energy: spiritual, mental, emotional, and physical. It also includes some examples of the ways we withdraw and deposit energy in our mind-body energy bank account.

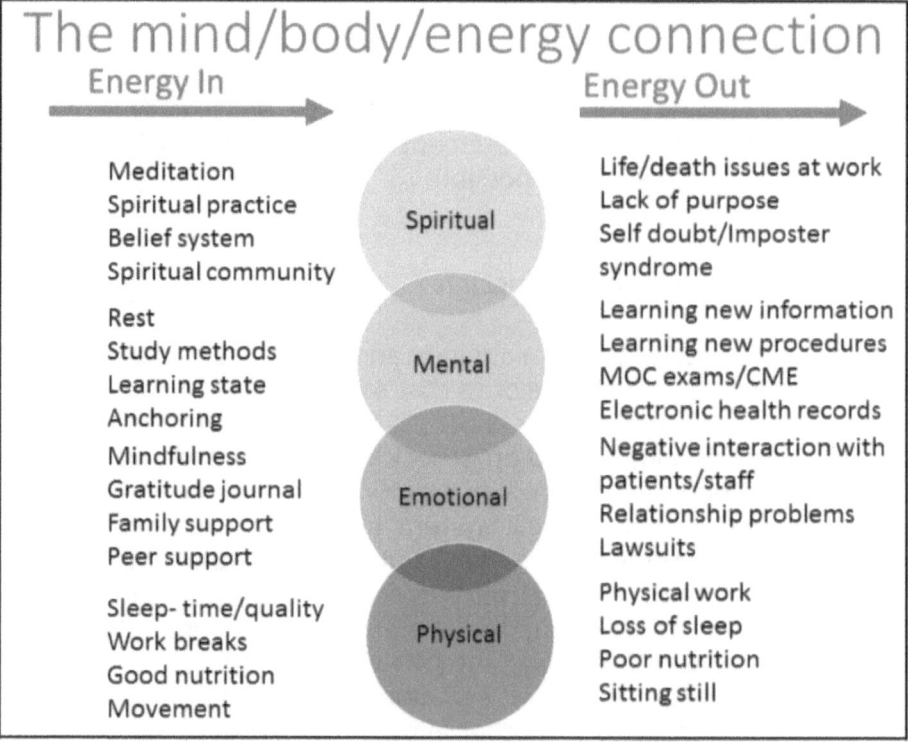

The mind/body/energy connection

Energy In →   **Energy Out** →

Energy In	Sphere	Energy Out
Meditation Spiritual practice Belief system Spiritual community	Spiritual	Life/death issues at work Lack of purpose Self doubt/Imposter syndrome
Rest Study methods Learning state Anchoring	Mental	Learning new information Learning new procedures MOC exams/CME Electronic health records
Mindfulness Gratitude journal Family support Peer support	Emotional	Negative interaction with patients/staff Relationship problems Lawsuits
Sleep- time/quality Work breaks Good nutrition Movement	Physical	Physical work Loss of sleep Poor nutrition Sitting still

Try this:

Use the following blank worksheet to evaluate your own energy balance. List the biggest energy drains in each part of your energy bank account on the right. Include work, home and other activities. Don't forget the energy vampires (people or situations that suck the life out of you.)

Then consider how you replenish your energy bank account. Include all the ways, people and activities in each area on the left.

Look at both lists. If you could eliminate one energy drain on the right list that would make the most difference to you, which one would it be? Circle it. What is the first thing you could do this week to eliminate it?

If you could maximize your energy replenishment, which activity/person on the left list would make the most difference in your life? Circle it. What is the first thing you could do this week to maximize it?

Energy In →		Energy Out →
1. _____		1. _____
2. _____	Spiritual	2. _____
3. _____		3. _____
1. _____		1. _____
2. _____	Mental	2. _____
3. _____		3. _____
1. _____		1. _____
2. _____	Emotional	2. _____
3. _____		3. _____
1. _____		1. _____
2. _____	Physical	2. _____
3. _____		3. _____

The four pillars of well-being

Four main pillars support our physical and mental well-being and longevity: **sleep, nutrition, physical activity,** and **community**, or positive interactions with our families, friends, and peers.

Sleep is perhaps the most important of these pillars. The average American today gets about two hours less sleep per night than they did 50 years ago. This is due to many factors including increased working hours and increased stimulation from television, internet, and smartphone usage. Sleep deprivation doesn't just result in significant cognitive impairment. It also leads to poor nutritional choices such as binge eating or snacking, and also has consequences that affect every area of our health—including decreasing insulin sensitivity, increasing gut permeability, increasing systemic inflammation, and decreasing immune function.

The second major pillar is **nutrition**. What we eat not only determines our physical health and our longevity, but along with sleep is a major factor contributing to our energy, mood, and even cognitive abilities.

The third pillar is **activity** or movement. By this, I don't necessarily mean exercising or working out at the gym. Simply getting up and moving from place to place or being active at work or around the house is critical for maintaining health as well as good mental and emotional functioning. Episodic vigorous physical activity (i.e., daily workouts) alone is not enough to maintain health and longevity if you are sedentary the rest of the time. Studies have shown that people who spend most of their time sitting have a much higher incidence of heart disease and early death.

The fourth pillar is **positive human interaction** or community. This requires communication, positive regard, and emotional supportiveness. Social isolation is a major factor in anxiety, depression, and physical illness.

Let's take a closer look at each of the pillars and discuss some ways we can improve in each area.

Sleep

The relationship between sleep and health seems so obvious you probably wonder why I'm even talking about it. Yet how many of us get eight hours of quality sleep a night? On the other hand, how many of you stay late after your shift or work back-to-back shifts either to help someone out or to make more money? How often do you put in more work hours after dinner, or stay up late to watch TV or use your computer—and then find that even after you go to bed, you have a hard time settling your mind and your body to fall asleep?

Studies have shown that the average adult needs approximately eight hours plus or minus 30 minutes of sleep per night in order to function optimally. However, the average American gets just six hours and 15 minutes of sleep on weeknights, and more than 30% of adult workers sleep *less* than six hours per weeknight. Lack of sleep is the single greatest risk factor for burnout on the job. Sleep deprivation also results in lower quality of work and decreased productivity.

Our attitude towards sleep is partially cultural and partly individual. Oftentimes, we think that working late or coming in early, even at the expense of our sleep time, makes us look more industrious and productive when the opposite is true. College students often take great pride in pulling "all-nighters" in order to study for an examination the next day; yet studies have shown that resting immediately after studying, even if only for an hour or two, results in improved recall the next day. Prior to the advent of medical student and resident work hour restriction, it was not unusual to work 36 hours on, 12 hours off, for weeks at a time. The idea was that trainees would get so much experience in performing their duties while sleep deprived that they would be able to do what they needed to so well that they could "do it in their sleep." Fortunately, that type of training has partially disappeared in light of the findings that sleep deprivation not only results in poorer learning, but also in poorer patient care and a negative patient experience. You can put yourself in your patient's shoes the next time you fly somewhere. Ask yourself how you would feel knowing that your pilot had just finished a 36-hour shift and had your life in his (sleep-deprived) hands!

Missing sleep can not only affect the next day, but the entire next week. I recently took a trip back from Europe to the United States where, due to timing, I lost an entire night's worth of sleep. I had to literally drag myself around for the first two days, and it took me a full five days of getting adequate sleep before I recovered my usual state of physical and mental functioning. You may think that getting just one night of insufficient sleep won't affect you, or that you might feel normal the next day. But the science tells us that losing even 90 minutes of sleep reduces alertness the next day over 25%. Even if you don't notice it, other people around you do, either in your performance or in your behavior. Clearly, it's crucial to make getting adequate sleep every night your first priority in avoiding burnout and maintaining your health. Because that's often easier said than done, let's discuss some strategies for doing so.

How to get a great night's sleep

I hope I've convinced you of the importance of getting a great night's sleep in order to have a great next day, maintain your health and avoid burnout. Below are some tips on how to get an optimal night sleep.

1. Go to bed at the same time every night if possible and get up about the same time the next day. Your body has an internal clock programmed in the neuroendocrine system. If you constantly change the time when you sleep, that internal clock doesn't work very well. Having said that, some people are early to bed, early to rise people, and some are night owls. Know your own internal rhythms and make sure to schedule out enough time that you can get eight hours of quality sleep.

2. Use the bedroom only for sleeping and sex. Your mind-body develops behavior triggers based on environmental cues and you want the bedroom to be associated with sleeping, not with snacking or watching TV.

3. Prepare to go to sleep beginning two hours before the time you intend to fall asleep.

During those two hours before bedtime, reduce the level of lighting in your house. As much as possible, avoid blue light sources such as cell phones, computer screens, and televisions. If you must use electronic devices, see if yours has a feature that reduces blue wavelengths or buy a pair of blue blocking glasses.

4. Avoid eating or vigorous exercising for two hours before going to bed. Your body has a hard time going abruptly from a high metabolic state to a low metabolic state like sleeping. There are some teas such as chamomile, kava or other non-caffeinated beverages which may be soothing to mind and body. Avoid caffeinated teas or coffee for two hours before going to bed. Some nutritional supplements such as melatonin are thought to help induce sleep. Of course, don't take any supplements which are medically contraindicated.

5. Make your bedroom dark and cold. For most people, the best sleeping conditions are in a dark room with no lights shining in or any visible indicator lights on electronic devices. If you can't make the room dark, you may consider wearing a sleep mask. A cool room (66 to 68 degrees) will help slow your metabolic rate and allow you to sleep more deeply.

6. If there are noises that disturb you, you may try wearing earplugs or using a white noise generating machine to mask any background sounds.

7. There are some techniques which may help settle the mind. One of these is journaling about something positive that happened that day and writing about a goal or something you're looking forward to the next day. Sometimes, if you have things on your mind that you must do the next day, it may be helpful to have a small pad of paper by your bed. You can make a list and then put those things aside mentally and physically by putting away the pad of paper. Deepak Chopra recommends a practice he calls recapitulation, which means reviewing in your mind your entire day from beginning to end

in just a minute or two. You can even do this in conjunction with your journaling.

Just to give you an idea of how this might go, I'll share with you my own sleep routine. I like to go to bed at about 9:30 every night and get up around 6:00 or 6:30 because I do my best work in the morning. For an hour before bed, I may read or listen to a book on my iPod to settle my mind. I do a quick journal entry before I brush my teeth and wash my face. Because I sleep with someone who likes a warmer room and I prefer a cooler environment, I have a device called a mattress chiller, which is a cooling water pad that fits underneath my mattress cover and allows me to control the temperature of my sleeping environment. This device has a small fan for cooling, which provides nice background white noise. It also generates negative ions in the air, which may promote relaxation and positivity. Once I'm in bed, I do 20 minutes of *yoga nidra*, which is a wonderfully relaxing body scan. Then I turn off the light and I'm usually asleep in 10 minutes or less.

You can use any of these suggestions to make your own bedtime routine. I'll talk about the easy way to start any new habit, including sleep habits in the next section. Remember, **a great day begins with a great night's sleep.**

Eat

How often have you skipped a meal because you're working so hard, and then grabbed a cookie or some other sugary snack to give yourself that energy boost to get through the rest of the day? Have you noticed how your mind and body feel an hour after eating that emergency junk food? Are you physically more energized, or do you actually feel *more* tired? Are you mentally clear or foggy?

You've probably noticed how hunger affects not only your clarity of mind, but also your mood. That's why proper nutrition is the second pillar of energy management. I purposely put this section after the section on the importance of sleep because getting adequate sleep is at the foundation of proper nutrition.

It's not just the amount of sleep that we get that counts, but the quality and time at which we sleep. Unfortunately, those of us who work in the medical professions may be forced work shifts that aren't conducive to a good sleep schedule. Working 12-hour shifts or being on night call—or worse yet, working a night shift regularly—wreaks havoc with our circadian rhythms, which govern not only our sleep but also our digestion. In addition, we are more likely to make bad decisions about what food to eat when we're sleep deprived. Conversely, what and when we eat has an effect on our sleep cycles. This can easily become a vicious circle where sleep deprivation causes us to seek highly processed, carbohydrate rich foods, which themselves may interrupt our sleep cycles.

What to eat

All of us in the healthcare professions encounter patients or clients with metabolic syndrome and type 2 diabetes. These diseases are so common today that life expectancy in the United States is now starting to decrease due to the related complications. We also know that most cases of type 2 diabetes are a consequence of years of poor food choices. It's no coincidence that this rampant epidemic of metabolic syndrome and type 2 diabetes coincided with the increase in amount and availability of processed foods—and their enormous load of refined carbohydrates over the last 50 years. In addition to their absence of nutritional value, another problem with these types of food is that the refined carbohydrates directly stimulate the dopamine mediated reward center in the brain. This is what makes them addictive, and what sets up a vicious cycle of cue-craving-response-reward and perpetuates an unhealthy eating habit.

It's ironic that medical professionals spend so much of our time dealing with diseases caused by poor nutritional habits, yet at the same time exhibit some of those habits and behaviors ourselves. Wouldn't it be great to be able to be able to counsel our patients on good nutrition through our *own* experience and to set a good example for them? I don't believe in a one-size-fits-all nutritional recommendation, but common sense and medical knowledge tells us that it's best to avoid a diet that results in wild swings in blood glucose, or even worse, prolonged elevation of blood glucose and development of insulin resistance.

There is a lot of scientific evidence about how our diet affects not only our health, but our performance, energy level, and mood. If you love the science, I recommend the book *Wired to Eat* by Robb Wolf. If the science doesn't turn you on, you can skip the book and read this summary of the findings and recommendations, which coincidentally are the same recommendations that my mother gave me growing up. Your diet should consist of primarily fresh fruits, vegetables including root vegetables, nuts and lean sources of protein including chicken, seafood, and lean cuts of beef or pork. Because so many people (including me) have a negative reaction to large loads of gluten and dairy products, these should be eaten sparingly. High-quality fats including olive oil, avocado oil (or avocados) and coconut oil are great for cooking and add both flavor and "mouth feel" to food.

So how do you handle your busy schedule and still eat high quality, nutritious foods and avoid the highly processed unhealthy foods that are so readily available? The best way is to prepare your own meals at home using high-quality natural ingredients that you purchase yourself. If you don't have the time or inclination to shop and cook, there are a variety of services that can deliver ingredients with instructions or even completed meals with healthful ingredients. Look online for suppliers local to you.

Eating out is more of a challenge, but if you follow the guidelines, you can find good choices on many restaurant menus, even in some fast food restaurants. Just watch out for hidden sugar, salt, and saturated fats that often come with restaurant meals. For specific recommendations, I refer you to Robb Wolf's book or website (https://robbwolf.com/) for additional resources.

Snacking at work or eating to deal with tiredness or low energy is a real challenge because you want something satisfying and close at hand. Unfortunately, what is usually close at hand is large variety of highly processed carbohydrate-rich junk food as well as sugary drinks. One way to avoid being sucked into this trap is to always have with you some healthy snacks such as whole fruit or nuts. One of the snacks I find most satisfying is an apple or a few peeled baby carrots and individual packets of high-quality almond butter, which is available in most health food stores. Individual containers of hummus and guacamole are also great if you have a refrigerator available at work. Having items such as these in arm's reach will help you make good nutritional choices instead of bad ones. If you have a cache of unhealthy snacks at work, give them away or put them in a place where they're hard to access so that you're less likely to make that choice in a weak moment.

Move

Until the last hundred years, our ancestors spent much of their time moving around on foot and doing physical labor like hunting, cultivating, finding and maintaining shelter, and raising children. All of this began to change with the advent of the Industrial Revolution. With the availability of electricity and artificial lighting, indoor work such as manufacturing increased. As cars became plentiful and cheap, the amount of physical activity required to move from place to place decreased dramatically. Now as more work has become computer-based and entertainment has been centered on television, the internet, and smartphones, the number of people leading very sedentary lifestyles has increased dramatically. But the human body was built to move, not to sit for long periods of time. As a result, we are now seeing the result of this inactivity in the skyrocketing rates of obesity and diabetes with all the attendant medical complications of those diseases.

It is now estimated that the average American spends more time sitting down (9.5 hours) than they do sleeping. Studies have shown that prolonged sitting by itself is an independent risk factor for development of heart disease and greater risk of death from any cause. Even an hour a day of vigorous physical activity is not enough to offset the risk of prolonged sitting or inactivity. Studies have shown that after two hours of sitting, your baseline metabolic activity drops by about 90% and HDL cholesterol (the good cholesterol) drops by 20%. That is why the rate of cardiovascular disease among deskbound workers is twice that of people who are active at work.

So, if you have a job, as I did, that requires sitting in front of a computer for eight to nine hours a day, how do you maintain your activity? The key is to break up those periods of sitting by periods of activity including standing, walking, stretching, or otherwise moving around and using your large muscle groups. Since it is well known that you can't maintain mental focus for a period greater than 40 to 60 minutes anyway, make it a habit to get up and move around for at least five minutes of every hour.

Also, try to build activity into your daily schedule. For example, park the car farther away from your work than usual and walk to your office. Try taking the stairs instead of using the elevator. When you want to talk to somebody, get up and go to their office instead of calling them on the phone or messaging them. Walk with your spouse, a friend, or your dog on a regular basis, and you will *all* feel better.

If you're a person who carries their smartphone with them, use the step-counter that's built into most smartphones or get a wristwatch that has a step counter in it. Try to make sure that you take at least 10,000 steps per day. It might sound like a lot, but I found that by being active at work, I was usually able to accumulate greater than 6,000 steps just by moving around. I finished the last 4,000 by working around the house and taking my dog for a walk in the evening. Just keeping track of the number of steps you take every day will result in improvement. As the saying goes, "That which gets measured improves."

Although weight-bearing exercise and going to the gym are not a substitute for general activity, they are very useful in their own right. Building muscle mass increases your basal metabolic rate and makes it easier to maintain a healthy weight. Studies have shown that even elderly people in their 80s and 90s are able to build muscle mass, and this activity increases their longevity. Other types of physical activity, such as yoga or other body work, can be extremely beneficial not only because they are a form of exercise—but because they also develop strength, flexibility, and balance which are important to your health and safety, particularly as you get older. Maintaining or improving your spinal and body alignment through yoga, tai chi, or similar activities helps reduce your risk for developing degenerative changes of the spine and joints as well.

Exercise or movement has mental and emotional benefits as well. Studies in students have shown that even 20 to 30 minutes of moderate exercise resulted in improved mood 2, 4, and even 24 hours later, as well as enhancing their creativity and memory recall.

Work-life harmony

Just as human beings did not evolve being sedentary, the need for social interaction is part of our ancestral makeup. Even with all the communication devices at our disposal nowadays, social isolation, anxiety and depression are epidemic. Studies have shown that inadequate social interaction and support is as great a risk to your health as smoking a pack of cigarettes per day. Studies with both monkeys and of children raised in orphanages in Eastern Europe have shown that absence of social interaction and support results in emotional, mental, and even physical stunting.

This makes sense if you look at how human beings evolved. Early hunter-gatherers lived in tight-knit social groups revolving around the family or tribe. Although social interactions weren't always positive, just the emotional and physical contact itself was wired into our brains. This kind of contact not only stimulates specific areas of the brain; it also releases specific hormones and neuroregulators that induce a feeling of closeness and counteract the neuroendocrine effects of stress.

As medical professionals, we often have so many professional obligations that we often put our social and family needs on the back burner. But interacting with people on Facebook, via text and even on the phone is no substitute for direct interaction. There is a lot of information out there about work-life balance. It is my opinion that achieving **work-life balance is essentially impossible for a medical**

professional. A truly balanced day would mean eight hours at work, eight hours at home or with friends, and eight hours of sleeping. I prefer to aim for **work-life harmony** or just **life harmony,** since work and life are inseparable. As in music, we achieve harmony by maximizing our flexibility within the constraints of the system. Here are some suggestions that I have gathered from others and from my own life.

Boundaries

There are different types of boundaries you can establish in your life. In the medical field, we must consider ethical and legal boundaries; but you also have to have personal boundaries related to your own values, goals, and life situation. By now, you have explored your own values and emotions as well as your communication skills through the other chapters in his book. In addition, once you've been practicing mindfulness regularly, you should be calmer and less stressed. This will allow you to discover what behavioral boundaries are important to you at work and at home. You first need to be clear with *yourself* about what your boundaries are before you can be clear with other people. Once you are clear with yourself, you need to enforce those boundaries politely, but firmly and consistently. It might take some repeated effort, but other people will respect you more. You'll also respect yourself and will be generally more satisfied with your life.

The second type of boundary is between different parts of your day. When you leave your house in the morning, that's a boundary. When you arrive at your workplace, that's another boundary. Arriving at home at the end of the day and spending some quiet time before bed are also boundaries you can observe. **Boundary rituals** are routine activities that you do when you cross one of those daily boundaries. The **single breath meditation** taught to me by Thich Nhat Hanh is a great boundary ritual that increases your mindfulness and lets you be fully present in the moment and emotionally available to the people you care about. To do this, take a deep breath into your abdomen then allow it to fully release as you think to yourself, "With this breath, I let go of everything else and come back fully to the present moment." Other boundary rituals include something as simple as changing your clothes. For example, changing from street clothes to scrubs at work, to gym clothes when you exercise, and to comfortable leisure clothes when you come home can help you move from one state of mind to the next. By observing these boundary rituals, you can feel more grounded, satisfied and aware of your work-life harmony.

The calendar hack

Events you plan are like goals. If you don't write them down, they're less likely to happen. You need to carve out time on your calendar to spend your friends, spouse or partner, children, and even time by yourself. You should have these times scheduled out on your calendar at least a week ahead of time. I call this the **calendar hack** and here's how I do it. I use Google Calendar because I find it to be simple and flexible and because I can access this calendar from my phone, tablet, or computer at any time. I have two separate Google accounts and two separate calendars: one for my personal use and one for my professional life. A single click or tap allows me to see either one separately or both superimposed.

First, I enter my appointments for the week on my professional calendar. If you have set hours of work and specific nights of call, you can put those intervals on your calendar without individual appointments. Then I go to work on my personal calendar. First, I put on social obligations and non-work-related meetings or classes. Then I talk to my partner and we decide on together one night a week when we will spend time with each other, going to dinner or a movie or a concert or something else that we both enjoy. I put those "date nights" on the calendar. If there are tickets involved, I purchase them to give myself extra motivation and commitment to make sure that it happens. You might not be able to schedule an evening every week with your spouse or partner, but you should have an evening **at least once every other week** and commit to spending that time with them. When you have your date night, make sure that you plan at least one more date night in the next two weeks.

Family time is just as important as personal time or date night. Again, I use Google Calendar and we have a separate calendar for the family.

When I still had family at home, we had a family meeting once a week where we put all family events including school, sports, and family social events on the family calendar. The owner of the family calendar (at that time, my wife) would send me an invitation via Google Calendar to any family events that were important for me to attend. These invitations would show up on my personal calendar or email and I could click "accept" and it would automatically appear on my combined calendar.

Just as with date night, it is very important to schedule out family time every week. In my house, family time revolved around Sunday afternoon and Sunday dinner. It was understood that attendance was expected by all family members and that we would do something that we all enjoyed. This was also the time when we set our family calendar for the next week. One of the major advantages of having a calendar where you can see your work, family and personal events all at the same time is it prevents you from overbooking yourself and can help you enforce your boundaries at work. For example, when one of my partners would ask me to cover their call rotation on a certain day, I could check my combined calendar. If I saw a conflict with an important personal or family event, I would simply say, "I'm very sorry, but I have another commitment at that time." It's very important when enforcing your boundaries to be very clear and kind; however, you do not have to justify yourself or explain your reasons.

The final part of achieving work-life harmony is taking adequate vacations to get away from work and spend time with your family or people outside of work. Regardless of the number of weeks of vacation that I had, I always made it a practice to take at least half of my vacation time with the family and the other half just with my partner or with my friends doing something that we enjoyed. Just as with date night or family time, you need to put these weeks on the calendar as far in advance as possible. Buy the tickets, pay for the cruise—do whatever you need to do to commit yourself financially and emotionally to making sure that it happens. Once it's on the calendar and it's paid for, it makes it much easier to enforce your boundaries regarding your time off.

Try this:

1. If you carry your cell phone with you, use the step counter app or get a watch with a step counter and keep track of your steps every day for a normal working week. Make a note of your average daily step count for that week. If it is less than 10,000 steps/day, increase your daily step count by 10% each week until you average 10,000 steps per day.

2. If you work sitting down most of the time, set a timer and get up and move around or walk somewhere for at least 5 minutes every hour.

3. Bring at least l healthy snack to work per day, such as an apple or some precut raw vegetable and some protein like a single pack of almond butter or cheese and eat it when you feel like a snack between meals.

4. In addition to your 5-15 minutes of sitting meditation per day, do the single breath meditation in your car before you enter your workplace. Do another one before you enter your home. What other routine activities could you use to remind you to do a single breath meditation?

5. Make a specific appointment for a "date night" with your spouse, partner, or a close friend within the next 2 weeks and commit to it. Plan something fun that you both enjoy. When you have your date night, make an appointment for the next one.

Key Points:

1. Getting about 8 hours of quality sleep per night is the foundation of your physical and mental health.

2. Quality nutrition is the second pillar of your physical and mental health and is dependent on getting adequate sleep.

3. Make it a habit to stand and move as much as you can during the day, even if you have to set a timer and/or modify how you do your work. Prolonged sitting is a risk factor for heart disease and early mortality and undermines the benefits of good nutrition and sleep.

4. You may not be able to achieve work-life balance, but you can achieve work-life harmony through creativity and flexibility.

5. Know your personal boundaries and enforce them consistently.

6. In-person social interaction is critical to good health and longevity. Even using some of the above suggestions will contribute to a feeling of harmony in your life.

References:

Shanafelt, Tait D. et al. Changes in Burnout and Satisfaction With Work-Life Integration in Physicians and the General US Working Population Between 2011 and 2017 Mayo Clinic Proceedings, Volume 94, Issue 9, 1681 - 1694

Wolf, Robb. Wired to Eat. Potter/Ten Speed/Harmony/Rodale. Kindle Edition. 2017

Rath, Tom. Eat Move Sleep: How Small Choices Lead to Big Changes. Missionday, LLC. Kindle Edition. 2013

AFTERWORD

Thank you for purchasing this book either in print form or eBook form. Part of the profits from the sale of the book go toward educating and training medical students and other healthcare trainees in the art of effective communication and the all-important skill of self-care.

Whether you read the book in its entirety, read individual chapters, or skimmed the entire work, I hope that you have found some hidden gems that will enable you to avoid burnout. If you are already burned out, I hope that some of the exercises and other learnings in this book enable you to not only recover, but to flourish and thrive in your healthcare occupation. One of the greatest tragedies of the burnout epidemic in healthcare is that so many professionals are leaving the field early and that young people often choose not to pursue a career in healthcare due to increasing stress and decreased reimbursement.

I believe that choosing a career in healthcare, whether as a physician, nurse, therapist, social worker, PA or MA, is still a good choice for many people despite the current dysfunctions of the system. There can be no more noble calling than caring for the health and well-being of another person. You just have to remember the warning that is printed on the card found in every airplane seatback: "Before attempting to assist other people, put your own oxygen mask on first."

So, it doesn't matter which of the tips or techniques from this book that you decide to apply in your own life. What's most important is that you **start now**. Even the smallest step is a step in the right direction that can ultimately lead you to a satisfying life of purpose and meaning.

To your health and well-being,

Gideon Strich, M.D.